KV-262-104

DRUGS NOT MENTIONED IN THE TEXT. It is not intended to give a complete list of additions to the B.P. 1958 of drugs not mentioned in this book, but the following are included, although in the interests of space they were omitted from the text.

Acetazolamide

Amylobarbitone

Atropine Methonitrate

Chloraquine Sulphate Injection

Diphtheria and Pertussis Vaccine

Diphtheria, Tetanus, and Pertussis Vaccine

Human Gamma Globulin

Hyaluronidase

Mustine Hydrochloride

Oxytetracycline and Procaine Injection

Paramethadione

Procainamide Hydrochloride

Procyclidine Hydrochloride

Propyliodone

Sodium Chloride and Dextrose Injection

Sodium Radiophosphate (^{32}P) Solution

Suxamethonium Bromide

Tetracycline and Procaine Injection

Zinc Undecenoate

AN INTRODUCTION TO PHARMACOLOGY AND THERAPEUTICS

AN INTRODUCTION TO
PHARMACOLOGY AND
THERAPEUTICS

BY

J. A. GUNN, C.B.E.
M.A., M.D., D.Sc., F.R.C.P.
Emeritus Professor of Pharmacology an
Therapeutics, University of Oxford

NINTH EDITION

WITH THE ASSISTANCE OF

J. D. P. GRAHAM
B.Sc., M.D., F.R.F.P.S.Glasg., F.R.C.P.Edin.
Senior Lecturer in Pharmacology
Welsh National School of Medicine, Cardiff

LONDON
OXFORD UNIVERSITY PRESS
1958

Oxford University Press, Amen House, London E.C.4

GLASGOW NEW YORK TORONTO MELBOURNE WELLINGTON
BOMBAY CALCUTTA MADRAS KARACHI KUALA LUMPUR
CAPE TOWN IBADAN NAIROBI ACCRA

© *Oxford University Press, 1958*

First edition 1929
Second edition 1931
Third edition 1932
Fourth edition 1934
Fifth edition 1936
Sixth edition 1940
Seventh edition 1944
Eighth edition 1948
Ninth edition 1958

PRINTED IN GREAT BRITAIN

PREFACE TO THE NINTH EDITION

THE thirty years which have elapsed since the first edition of this book was published have been a period of unparalleled advances in Pharmacology and Therapeutics. The discovery of new remedies has revolutionized the treatment of disease. Research laboratories, academic and commercial, have multiplied the world over, and investigation proceeds with gathering momentum. New chemical compounds are being prepared and pharmacologically tested in their hundreds. Only a very few merit therapeutic trial and still fewer succeed in finding an assured place in medical practice.

The medical practitioner finds it hard to keep up with these rapid and continuous advances. The student beginning the subject is faced with a formidable list of outlandish names with which he must learn to associate pharmacological and therapeutical properties. The writer of an introductory book must discriminate in his choice of material. For this, fortunately, the current editions of the British and United States Pharmacopoeias provide a reliable general guide.

I have been stimulated to revise this little book by requests from teachers and from the Oxford University Press, and in its final completion have had valued help from my old colleague, Dr. J. D. P. Graham. All chapters have been revised and most of them largely rewritten. Some new sections have been added. Of groups of drugs, perhaps the most substantial additions have been made to antibiotics, hormones, autonomic drugs, anaesthetics, analgesics, sedatives, and antihistamines. I hope that as revised the book may continue to fulfil its original purpose.

J. A. G.

Hermitage, Berks.
August 1957

PREFACE TO THE FIRST EDITION

DURING the years in which I have had the privilege of teaching medical students in Oxford, I have given a course of lectures dealing with the actions and uses of drugs, supplemented by practical courses in Pharmacology and in Pharmacy. Owing to the increasing demands upon the medical curriculum, this yearly course of lectures has been limited to fifty. Such a course could not give much more than a general sketch of the subject, the student being left to fill in detail from text-books or other sources. Without such a general survey the student is apt to lose himself in a mass of detail and often fails to get any sense of proportion or scheme of classification.

I have often wished to alter this procedure by providing the student with such a short but comprehensive survey in book form as would leave the lecturer more freedom and latitude to deal with more advanced and advancing aspects of the subject. The smaller books that are available do not furnish the desired survey because they achieve brevity by compression rather than by selection and arrangement. I am also frequently asked to recommend a book which a student can read in the vacation before attending lectures, and for this a large text-book is unsuitable.

It is for these purposes that this little book has been written, though I can hardly hope that its sphere of usefulness will be commensurate with the time I have spent upon its compilation.

J. A. G.

Oxford 1929

CONTENTS

*Were angels to write books, they would
never write folios*

OLIVER GOLDSMITH

I

INTRODUCTION

ORIGIN AND SOURCES OF DRUGS

ALL races of mankind have tried to heal those who suffer from diseases, and of the many curative methods which have been employed, one of the most ancient and successful has been treatment by means of drugs. The drugs which are used medicinally at the present day have been discovered at different times and in different countries. They come from different sources; animal, vegetable, and mineral substances, as well as artificially prepared compounds, have all been pressed into service as remedial agents.

It is not difficult to imagine how, for example, plants came to be used as remedies. Man had to discover which plants were edible and which were not. They bore no labels. In the process of seeking for food, it would be found that some plants produce unusual effects. They might purge, for example, and the step would be a fairly easy one to use such a plant as a remedy for constipation. Some would be found to be powerful poisons, and extracts of these came to be used in some countries, for example, as arrow poisons. Long before there was any science of experimental pharmacology, or even before there was any real knowledge of the causes of disease, a large amount of information had thus accrued of the remedial and toxic properties of plants.

One can imagine also how an elementary knowledge of pharmaceutical processes would arise. A recognition of any unusual action of a plant might result at first from eating a leaf. A leaf stored for future use might crumble, and it would be found that the leaf retained its activity in the form of a powder. If it were cooked, it might be noticed that the active properties of the plant were conveyed to the water in which the plant was cooked, and even to the residue left when the water evaporated. So might come about the employment of plants in the form of a powder, an infusion, or an extract, methods of preparation which are still in use.

It required a much greater knowledge (in some cases a very modern knowledge) of chemistry to determine which particular constituent of a plant was responsible for its curative or toxic actions, and to determine the chemical nature of this, the 'active principle' as it is called. This kind of knowledge has really been acquired only in the last century. For example, cinchona bark was used as a remedy for malaria for about two centuries before the active principle, quinine, was isolated from it. The active principles of most important medicinal plants are now known, and in some cases their exact chemical composition. Especially in the last fifty years it has become possible with advancing knowledge to use the active principles in place of a crude drug or of extracts from it. The amount of active principle in a plant varies with such factors as the soil in which it grows and the climate. Even if an extract is always made in the same way, therefore, its activity will vary. But the active principle is a definite chemical substance, of unvarying composition and often more stable than an extract, and therefore dosage with it can be more accurate.

One large group of drugs, therefore, consists of plants or parts of them, of extracts made from plants, and of active principles—alkaloids, for example—isolated from plants. Other substances have been used as remedies. Some of these are substances occurring in nature like sulphur, compounds of iron, or salts like Epsom salts. A very important group of drugs has been introduced especially in the last half-century or so, substances which have been manufactured in the chemical laboratory. An early type of such a substance would be alcohol, manufactured by the fermentation of sugar. The important anaesthetics chloroform and ether are artificially made, so are most of the hypnotics, chloral and barbiturates for example. Though plant constituents continue to be investigated with a view to discovering new remedies, an increasing number of new drugs are such compounds artificially synthesized or manufactured in the chemical laboratory.

It follows from this that not only have drugs come to us from different sources and through different channels, but our knowledge of their action and effects has been variously acquired. Drugs were employed in the treatment of diseases long before the pathology of these diseases was understood. The investigation of the pharmacological actions of drugs is a comparatively new science. In the course of time, therefore, various remedial actions of drugs were discovered for which no scientific explanation could, at the time, be given. With the advances in knowledge of physiology, pathology, and pharmacology, especially in the last half-century, these explanations have in many cases been forthcoming. To make a rough classification, our present knowledge of the effects of drugs has been acquired in two ways. Older remedies were discovered chiefly by observing their remedial effects in diseases in man, while the pharmacological basis of these effects has only recently, and as yet imperfectly, been established. On the other hand, substances, artificial or other, which are now for the first time investigated as to their possible value as remedial agents, are first examined, usually on laboratory animals, as to their physiological actions and toxicity, and it is upon the results of this investigation that a possible field for their tentative therapeutic use is based.

Pharmacology (Greek, *pharmakon*, a drug) may be defined as the action of drugs on normal animals or tissues. *Therapeutics* (Greek, *therapeuein*, to heal) means, so far as drugs are concerned, their remedial action in the treatment of disease. *Chemotherapy*, a word not precisely defined, generally refers to treatment by means of substances of known chemical composition, as opposed to antitoxins. From the experimental point of view, it differs from pharmacology in that the therapeutic action of a drug is usually investigated in animals infected with a specific pathogenic micro-organism.

The term *Pharmacognosy* is applied to the knowledge of the sources and chemical properties of drugs, while the art of preparing drugs in forms suitable for medicinal administration is called *Pharmacy*.

As a guide to the physician and pharmacist, most countries publish from time to time an authoritative list of drugs in general use with information regarding their sources and physico-chemical properties, doses, &c. It contains also a description of standard 'preparations' of drugs. A most important function of a pharmacopoeia is to lay down standards of composition and purity to which all medicaments used in regular practice should conform. As new drugs are introduced or old ones discarded, this list has to be revised. In this country the book in question is called the *British Pharmacopoeia* and it is published under the direction of the General Medical Council. Amendments to the current edition may be published in an *Addendum*, which has the same authority as the *British Pharmacopoeia*. The latest edition was published in 1953 and the *Addendum 1955 to the British Pharmacopoeia 1953* became official in 1956. Drugs or preparations recognized in this book are called 'official' remedies; or the initials (B.P.) are placed after the name of the drug. Similarly (U.S.P.) stands for the *Pharmacopeia of the United States*, the Fifteenth Revision of which was issued in 1955, (U.S.P. XV), and the first supplement in 1957. Another book, the *British Pharmaceutical Codex* (B.P.C.), published by direction of the Council of the Pharmaceutical Society of Great Britain, gives information mainly about medicaments which, though in fairly constant demand, are not included among official remedies. The current edition was published in 1954 and amendments are given in a supplement which is published between editions, the latest one being June 1957. It includes a large number of formulae and, unlike the *Pharmacopoeia*, descriptions of the actions and uses of drugs. The *British National Formulary 1957* gives a list of formulae useful in general medical practice especially under the National Health Scheme. It gives useful and concise information about the actions of some important groups of remedies. An alternative edition is now available in which the arrangement is on a pharmacological basis, for the use of medical students. The American *National Formulary* covers much the same ground as the B.P.C. *New and Nonofficial Remedies*, issued annually under the direction of the American Medical Association, gives helpful information about new drugs and their therapeutic values.

METHODS OF ACTION OF DRUGS AND CONDITIONS INFLUENCING THESE

LOCAL AND GENERAL ACTIONS

By local action is meant the action which a drug exerts at the site of application and before it is absorbed into the blood stream. This includes not only such obviously external actions as, for example, the action of an ointment on the skin or of a solution applied to the conjunctiva, but also the action of a gargle on the surface of the throat or of a solution used to wash out the bladder. Drugs administered by mouth act first on the surface of the alimentary canal, effects which are included among local actions.

By general action is meant the action of a drug *after absorption*. In this case the drug is carried by the blood to all the tissues in the body, which therefore are all subjected to the same concentration of it. It is found, however, that under these circumstances the different tissues of the body are not equally sensitive to the action of any drug. In other words, drugs have what is called a *selective action* on the tissues. This selective action is more marked with some drugs than with others, but is displayed by them all. Indeed, the possibility of their being used medicinally usually depends upon this. When a dose of 2 milligrams of strychnine is given intravenously to a man weighing 70 kilograms, the concentration in the blood (once it is evenly distributed and before any of it is excreted) is about 1 part in 2 or 3 millions. This concentration may stimulate the central nervous system, but even much larger doses, which would give correspondingly higher concentrations in the blood, have no such effect on other tissues. Extract of pituitary gland is extensively used to stimulate the contractions of the uterus in labour, but it could hardly be used for this purpose if it had an equal effect on the muscle of the bronchi, because in this case an undesirable attack of asthma would accompany the desired action on the uterus. It will be readily understood that one generally desires a drug to act primarily on one organ or system, and it is upon the fact that they usually do this— that they exhibit a selective action on particular organs—that the therapeutic use of drugs depends.

When strychnine acts on the central nervous system or pituitary extract on the uterine muscle, it may be presumed that there is some physical or chemical reaction between the drug and the tissue acted upon. As to the nature of such reactions we have scarcely any accurate knowledge. When one considers the complexity of the chemical structure, both of living cells and of many drugs, the fact that we cannot as yet explain the *interactions between living cell and drug* is not surprising. In the case of drugs of simpler constitution producing grosser actions, a chemical explanation can in some cases be given; for example, the caustic action of silver nitrate is due in part at least to the precipitation of the proteins of the cell by the silver ion. Recent work has shown that the action of drugs on enzymes may play a fundamental part in pharmacology, e.g. the action of physostigmine in inhibiting cholinesterase.

Though our knowledge of the reactions between cell and drug is as yet meagre, it has been found that substances of similar chemical constitution often produce similar pharmacological actions. When the structural composition of adrenaline was once determined, not only could adrenaline be manufactured synthetically in the laboratory, but other natural and artificial compounds having a similar chemical composition were found in many cases to exert physiological actions more or less similar to those produced by adrenaline. This kind of investigation into what is called the *relation between chemical composition and pharmacological action* has greatly increased pharmacological knowledge and added new and useful drugs.

When strychnine acts on the central nervous system, or in general when any drug acts on any organ, it cannot alter the normal functions of that organ. No drug can, for example, cause a nerve cell to contract rhythmically, or a cardiac cell to exhibit reflex action, or a salivary gland to secrete bile. All a drug can do is to increase or decrease the excitability of a nerve cell, change the rate or force of the heart's contractions, or make a salivary gland eliminate more or less of its normal secretion. In other words, *drugs can only change activities of organs quantitatively, not qualitatively*; but this quantitative change, combined with the selective action of drugs, is fortunately usually enough for our purpose. The fact that a drug can only increase or decrease the activities of an organ necessitates the continual description of pharmacological action as *stimulation* or *depression* of the activities of organs; but from what has been said it will be clear that from this reiteration there is no escape.

Two milligrams of strychnine injected into a man may produce a just measurable increase in the excitability of certain reflexes; 200 milligrams may cause death from violent convulsions. A small (therapeutic) dose of atropine may stimulate certain parts of the central nervous system, which will be paralysed by a larger dose of the same drug. Very weak concentrations of quinine may accelerate the movements of amoebae, whereas higher concentrations will arrest those movements. It is clear, therefore, that one cannot speak of the actions of a drug as something fixed. The degree of action always, and even sometimes the type of action, depend upon the dose or concentration. Seeing, therefore, that whenever a drug is intelligently prescribed it must be given with the intention of producing a definite effect, it would seem to be obvious that the question of dosage is all-important. And yet much of the doubt and confusion that still prevails regarding the pharmacological actions and therapeutic values of drugs is due to want of persistent recognition of this elementary fact. To the student beginning this subject, the task of learning doses is bound to be wearisome, but it may be some consolation to remember that the remedial value of a drug depends upon the dose of it that is given.

Very few drugs are devoid of harmful or toxic effects if given in sufficiently high dosage. An estimate of the factor of safety can be obtained from the *therapeutic index*. This is the ratio of the greatest amount that can be tolerated (or the least amount that will produce toxic effects) to the dosage which may reasonably be expected to exert the desired therapeutic effect. The greater this index the greater is the margin of safety in using a drug. Drugs vary widely in their therapeutic index, from e.g. d-tubocurarine in which it is little more than unity to penicillin in which it is very high. This means that it is difficult to get the desired effect from d-tubocurarine without dangerous symptoms occurring (though they can be counteracted) whereas with penicillin, apart from idiosyncrasy reactions (p. 9), the contrary is true.

For the guidance of the practitioner a pharmacopoeia, therefore, mentions the doses of drugs; the *British Pharmacopoeia* gives a minimum and maximum dose, whereas the *United States Pharmacopeia* gives the usual dose, and range. The pharmacopoeial dose is not authoritatively enjoined as binding upon prescribers but is intended for general guidance and represents, unless otherwise stated, the average range of quantities which are generally regarded as suitable for an adult when administered by mouth. The oral dose of many substances may be repeated three or four times in 24 hours. For some substances the doses mentioned are those given over a stated period, e.g. daily. If it is usual to administer a drug otherwise than by mouth, the dose suitable for that method is stated.

In experimental pharmacology, as in all scientific work, the metric system of weights and measures is now internationally employed, and there are clear advantages in using this system in practical therapeutics. The B.P. and the U.S.P. express all doses in the metric system but as the Imperial system has been long used in medical practice in English-speaking countries, the B.P. continues to give additionally in that system the doses of many substances and preparations which are still frequently prescribed in it. In the U.S.P. all doses below 1 gramme are expressed in milligrams, whereas the B.P. gives them as decimals of a gramme from 100 mg. (0·1 G.) upwards, except where the smaller of the two quantities given is less than

100 mg.: both amounts are then given in milligrams; (e.g. 60–300 mg.).

There are certain conditions influencing dosage which may be conveniently mentioned here. When a drug is given, for example, to produce some action after absorption, the amount of effect that it produces depends usually upon the concentration of the drug in the blood, and consequently upon the volume of the blood. As the volume of blood in an infant will be much less than that of an adult, a proportionately smaller dose will be required to produce the same concentration of the drug in the blood. If one regards the drug as evenly distributed through all the tissues, the general result will be the same. In animals of the same species, therefore, the dose of a drug required to produce a given effect ought to be roughly proportioned to *body weight*; and this is found to be the case, though, with some drugs especially, it may be more nearly proportional to body surface. In any case the dose for a child will depend upon its size and weight. It is not always convenient to weigh a child, and the estimation of the surface area of the body requires some mathematical calculation; but it is usually possible to obtain the age of the child, and as this bears some relation to size and weight, a rough estimate of dosage can be made on the basis of *age*. One simple formula for this, called Young's Formula, is to take the age divided by the age plus 12, which gives a fair average fraction of the adult dose which is suitable for a child. For example, a child of three would get three-fifteenths or one-fifth of the adult dose. By Clark's rule the fraction of the adult dose is given by the child's weight in pounds divided by 150.

Even with these precautions, however, and even if the dose be accurately measured in proportion to body weight, it will still be found that individuals vary in their reaction to drugs. A marked divergence from normal reaction is called *Idiosyncrasy*, which merely means any kind of peculiar reaction. An individual may show an excessive reaction to a normal dose (*Hypersusceptibility*), for example, infants are hypersusceptible to opium: or a diminished reaction (*Tolerance*), for example, children are very tolerant of salicylates: or an unusual reaction (idiosyncrasy proper), for example, a usual dose of quinine produces in a small proportion of people a severe nettle-rash.

The word *Allergy* is now in common use to signify an unusual response, either quantitative or qualitative, to a drug. Certain articles of food, for example, shellfish, may provoke an 'allergic' response in certain people. This tendency may apparently be inborn and similar unusual reactions may occur to a drug when it is taken for the first time; but they may also result only from repeated administration. Anaphylaxis (p. 262) is a form of allergy and some allergic responses to drugs may be fundamentally allied to it. Among the commoner symptoms are drug rashes and asthma.

Tolerance may be of two kinds. It may be inborn, in which case it is usually called *Natural Tolerance*; or it may be attained through repeated administration, in which case it is called *Acquired Tolerance*. The latter kind of tolerance is especially prone to occur with hypnotic drugs; a person, for example, who habitually indulges in morphine may come to withstand a dose which would kill several people who were unaccustomed to it. It is important to remember that acquired tolerance to drugs is usually, if not always, of a different nature from acquired immunity to proteins, toxins, or bacteria. In the latter case repeated administration induces the tissue cells to manufacture and shed off into the body fluids antibodies which neutralize or inactivate the foreign substance. Tolerance to drugs, however, is acquired in other ways; usually the body acquires an increased power of metabolizing or of excreting the drug, or the cells become, in some way not yet understood, more resistant to its action.

Differences in age, weight, susceptibility, &c., of patients cannot be avoided and have to be taken into account in dosage. But this care would avail little if a drug itself were liable to vary in activity or toxicity. One function of a pharmacopoeia is to lay down standards of purity and constancy of drugs. Generally this can be done by ordinary chemical methods. Thus both B.P. and U.S.P. require that Tincture of

Opium must contain 1 per cent. of anhydrous morphine (limits 0·95 to 1·05) and a *chemical assay* is prescribed whereby it can be determined whether any sample of Tincture of Opium satisfies these requirements. For certain drugs or preparations, however, usually because the active principles are not sufficiently known or cannot be quantitatively isolated, satisfactory chemical assays are not at present possible. These drugs, if accuracy of dosage is imperative, have to be assayed by a biological method.

A *biological assay* differs from a chemical assay in that the test depends on the measurement, not of some chemical or physical property but of some biological response. Such a response may, however, vary quantitatively even in animals of the same species. For a biological assay of adequate accuracy, it is, therefore, necessary: (1) to prepare an official standard preparation of the drug in sufficient quantity which can be kept under conditions in which its potency will remain unaltered, and (2) to compare by means of a measurable biological response, determined under scrupulously controlled conditions of experiment, the activity of the sample of the drug to be tested with that of the standard preparation. The biological response employed varies with the particular drug. Examples of official preparations requiring biological assay are digitalis, extracts of animal organs, for example insulin, and antitoxins.

METHODS BY WHICH DRUGS ARE ADMINISTERED

Before considering the action of drugs in detail, it may be well first to consider the chief channels by which drugs are administered, though some of these, being matters of common knowledge, will be already familiar.

For exerting any desired local actions, drugs can be applied directly to accessible surfaces, e.g. the skin, mucous membranes, wounds, &c.

To produce their general actions drugs may be given in any convenient way that will permit of their absorption. As a rule drugs are not easily absorbed from the skin but are much more readily absorbed from mucous membranes. The nasal mucous membrane, for example, absorbs many drugs rapidly. Many volatile substances can be very rapidly absorbed from the enormous surface of the lung alveoli; volatile general anaesthetics, for example, can thus be very conveniently given by *inhalation* (p. 94).

Naturally, one of the commonest methods of giving drugs is *by mouth*. This is the obvious method of administration when a local action on the alimentary canal is desired, but drugs can also be given by this channel with a view to their absorption. Drugs vary very much in the readiness with which they are absorbed from the alimentary canal. With the important exception of alcohol, few drugs are absorbed from the stomach; absorption occurs chiefly from the small intestine and occurs there in all degrees, ranging from the swift absorption of iodides to the almost complete inabsorbability of liquid paraffin. A frequent drawback to oral administration is that drugs may be chemically altered in the alimentary canal, or they may interfere with digestion. A drug likely to cause local irritation of the stomach should be given well diluted or after a meal, in which case the drug will be diluted with inert matter and less of it will have immediate contact with the mucuous membrane. This, however, will usually delay absorption because the drug will reach the intestine, where it can be absorbed, only *pari passu* with the rest of the stomach contents. More rapid absorption is likely to occur if a drug is given on an empty stomach because it will then pass more rapidly into the intestine. Substances exceptionally nauseating or irritant may be given in keratinized capsules which resist gastric digestion. Drugs may also be given *by rectum*, either for a local action on the lower bowel or with a view to absorption.

Either to avoid chemical change or merely for speed of action, drugs may be injected under the skin. As many substances, especially if soluble in the body fluids, are absorbed more rapidly from *subcutaneous injection* than from the intestine, while the rate of excretion is uninfluenced, the concentration of the drug in the blood is, as a general rule, temporarily higher with subcutaneous injection than with oral administration. The dose necessary to produce a given effect is therefore usually smaller; it varies in the case of different drugs. If a drug is likely to cause much pain if injected under the skin, it can be injected into a muscle instead. From such an *intramuscular injection*, drugs are, as a rule, more rapidly absorbed than from hypodermic injection, for the muscle is more vascular than the subcutaneous tissues. When it is imperative that a drug should enter the blood stream unaltered or immediately, or when it is too irritating to be given by mouth or subcutaneously, it may be given by *intravenous injection*. Injected into a vein, a drug exerts its full action often instantaneously, while the time afforded for excretion, as compared with the time of entering the blood, is negligible. The dose is usually correspondingly small and must be very accurate, and usually the drug should be injected slowly and well diluted. *Intrathecal injection* or administration directly into the cerebrospinal fluid is only resorted to in special cases where it is necessary to obtain an effective concentration of the agent without delay in the central nervous system. Few drugs which are of value in combating infection are capable of passing the blood-brain barrier. They are therefore ineffective when given by mouth or hypodermically.

All drugs given by injection have to be prepared in a stable, sterile, isotonic solution of accurately known concentration, free from pyrogens which might cause a febrile reaction.

PREPARATIONS OF DRUGS

As one might anticipate, for these different methods of administration drugs have to be prepared in different ways. In a medical 'prescription' the physician gives written directions to the dispensing chemist as to how a drug or combination of drugs is to be prepared for administration in a particular case. Often such a prescription may be very simple. For example, a drug, such as aspirin, which has a definite chemical composition and can be obtained pure, which has little taste and is given in a dose that can conveniently be weighed, may be prescribed as such—as a powder or tablet—in the requisite quantities. On the other hand, other drugs, especially parts of plants, may have to undergo a series of manipulations before they are in a condition suitable for administration. As the activity of a preparation will depend upon many varying factors and as it may take many hours to make and can be more economically done with a large bulk of material, it would be an obvious advantage if, instead of every physician ordering his own formula, a standard preparation could be used which would always be of the same strength and which the dispenser could have in stock ready for immediate use. This is what is actually done in the case of pharmacopoeial preparations.

The pharmacopoeia includes, therefore, not only drugs themselves, but a large number of such 'Preparations'. Some drugs require little else than an official tablet; others have several preparations. In this book only a selection of official preparations can be mentioned. The selection of particular preparations for inclusion in a pharmacopoeia is generally based upon two factors—the physical or chemical properties of a drug and the uses to which it is put.

The different types of pharmaceutical preparations come under the subject of Pharmacy, but the more important may be briefly mentioned here. They can be classified in part on the basis of their solubilities.

Water is frequently used as solvent, and the resulting preparations are differently named according to the process used. A solution of a non-volatile substance is called a *Solution* (*Liquor*); if the substance be volatile, a *Water* (*Aqua*). An *Infusion* is obtained by treating the prepared drug with (usually boiling) water and straining. A *Syrup* consists of a strong solution of cane-sugar in water, in which a drug may be dissolved.

Alcohol is used as a solvent in *Tinctures*, which are prepared in various ways. If the substance is volatile, the alcoholic solution is called a *Spirit*. In a *Glycerin*, B.P. (*Glycerite*, U.S.P.), the solvent is a mixture of glycerin and water.

Preparations can also be classified according to their method of administration. For oral administration solid substances can be given simply in the form of a *Powder* (Pulvis) or compressed into *Tablets* (Tabellae) or incorporated with some suitable excipient into the form of a *Pill*. In recent years a great change has come over dispensing practice in regard to the relative popularity of these three preparations. In the B.P. 1932 there were 7 official pills, 8 powders, and 1 tablet; in the B.P. 1953 no pill, 7 powders, and 62 tablets. Tablets can be made by machinery with sufficient uniformity in size and amount of drug. They are portable, keep well as a rule, and they are cheaper.

Extracts are made usually by dissolving out the active principles of plants in water or alcohol and subsequently evaporating the solution. They may be *Liquid Extracts* (B.P.), *Fluid Extracts* (U.S.P.), or *Dry Extracts*, according to the degree of evaporation of the solvent.

Substances may also be given by mouth in fluid form, generally called a *Mixture*. A mixture may contain substances in solution, suspension, or emulsion. They are in this way easily swallowed, and domestic measures of volume can be used for subdivision. In routine practice, therefore, drugs are frequently prescribed in mixtures.

Similar fluid preparations for injection into the rectum are called *Enemas*; while solid cylindrical bodies used for insertion into the rectum are called *Suppositories*, or *Pessaries* if for vaginal use.

The pharmacopoeias contain certain *Injections*, solutions or suspensions in a watery or oily vehicle, which require special preparation or special precautions in regard to sterility, &c.

For external application a drug may be incorporated with a fatty basis in an *Ointment* (Unguentum); if intended to be applied with friction, it can preferably have an oily or alcoholic basis, in which case the preparation is called a *Liniment*. A solid adhesive preparation for stationary application is called a *Plaster*.

Special preparations are often required for application to mucous surfaces, e.g. of the throat, eye, urethra, &c.; but these are usually made up as required, and few such preparations have as yet found their way into the pharmacopoeia. The B.P. contains, for example, *Eye Ointments* (Oculenta).

WEIGHTS AND MEASURES

METRIC SYSTEM

WEIGHTS

1 Kilogram (kg.)	= 1,000 grammes (G.)
1 Gramme (G.)	= 1,000 milligrams (mg.)
(Gm. in U.S.P.)	

VOLUMES

1 Litre (L.)	= 1,000 millilitres (ml.)

IMPERIAL SYSTEM

WEIGHTS

437·5 Grains (gr.)	= 1 ounce (avoirdupois) (oz.)
16 Ounces (7,000 gr.)	= 1 pound (lb.)

VOLUMES

60 Minims (min.)	= 1 fluid drachm (fl. dr.) (one tea-spoonful)
4 Fluid Drachms	= $\frac{1}{2}$ fluid ounce ($\frac{1}{2}$ fl. oz.) (one tablespoonful)
8 Fluid Drachms	= 1 fluid ounce (fl. oz.)
20 Fluid Ounces	= 1 pint (pt.)

RELATIONS OF METRIC AND IMPERIAL SYSTEMS

For converting doses in the Imperial System into doses in the Metric System, the following *approximate* equivalents will assist:

WEIGHTS

IMPERIAL			METRIC	
$\frac{1}{100}$ Grain =	0·6 milligrams	=	0·0006 gramme	
$\frac{1}{10}$,, =	6	,,	=	0·006 ,,
1 ,, = 60		,,	=	0·06 ,,
10 Grains			=	0·6 ,,
15 ,,			=	1 ,,
1 Ounce			=	30 grammes

VOLUMES

IMPERIAL		METRIC
1 Minim	=	0·06 ml. or c.c.
10 Minims	=	0·6 ,,
15 ,,	=	1 ,,
1 Fluid Drachm	=	4 ,,
1 Fluid Ounce	=	30 ,,

With regard to higher values it is useful to remember that 1 kg. = 2·2 pounds and conversely 1 pound = 454 grammes; 1 litre = 1·76 pints and conversely 1 pint = 0·568 litres.

THE FORM OF A PRESCRIPTION

In the writing of a medical prescription, in which the prescriber informs the pharmacist as to what preparation is to be supplied and how it is to be labelled with instructions for the patient, it is much to the advantage of both prescriber and dispenser that the prescription should adhere to a standard form. This saves time and prevents mistakes. Here it is only possible to indicate and illustrate the conventional way of setting out a prescription. When using Imperial Measure the use of symbols should be avoided where any possibility of confusion might arise.

Doctor's Address
Date

Patient's Name

Patient's Address

℞ Ammonium Bicarbonate	3 gr.
Sodium Bicarbonate	10 gr.
Tincture of Ipecacuanha	20 min.
Chloroform Water	to $\frac{1}{2}$ fl. oz.

Make a mixture and send 6 fl. oz.
Sig.: Take 1 tablespoonful 3 times a day after meals.

Doctor's Signature

This is similar to the MIXTURE OF IPECACUANHA, ALKALINE (Ipecacuanha and Alkali Mixture) of the B.P.C. and the *British National Formulary*. In it the sodium bicarbonate acts as an alkali, ammonium bicarbonate and ipecacuanha as expectorants and the chloroform water serves as a flavouring agent and provides the necessary bulk of fluid. The advantage of such a standard formula is that the prescriber need not write out the prescription in full but merely order IPECACUANHA AND ALKALI MIXTURE. B.P.C.

The 'Sig.' (signetur, 'let it be labelled') is the instruction to the patient to be written on the label, the ℞ part is instructions to the pharmacist as to what is to be dispensed.

If the metric system is used in prescribing, a vertical line should be drawn to indicate the place of the decimal points of the ingredients. If the prescription contains a drug controlled by the Dangerous Drugs Act, special regulations are enjoined upon both prescriber and pharmacist.

II

WATER AND SALTS

GENERAL PRINCIPLES

LIVING protoplasm may be regarded as a liquid, containing various colloids and crystalloids in solution. It is not homogeneous, like a solution of sodium chloride, but contains an immense number of particles in the colloidal state. In order to prevent indiscriminate diffusion of substances from the protoplasm into the surrounding medium, and to maintain the identity and integrity of the cell, the latter is surrounded by a limiting membrane. This membrane is generally believed to be composed of a complex colloidal mixture of proteins and lipoids; and is impermeable to colloids but permeable to substances soluble in lipoids. The permeability to salts, sugar, and water varies with different cells or even with the same cell in different states of functional activity. Most animal cells are, however, permeable to water and to some salts, and are therefore free to change their dimensions by giving up or absorbing water. In order that they may remain in a normal state, therefore, they must be surrounded by an isotonic medium, with which they keep in equilibrium. Most cells of the body may be regarded as surrounded by blood plasma or by lymph, these body fluids being a solution of proteins, salts, &c., in water. Unless there were some mechanism for keeping the composition and osmotic pressure of these fluids constant, the cells would be liable to continual changes in composition and in size. One of the functions of the kidneys is to maintain the constancy of these fluids in spite of the changes which would otherwise result from variations in the intake and output of water or salts. If there be an undue loss of water, e.g. by profuse sweating, the blood becomes more concentrated. This, among other effects, diminishes the secretions of the mouth and throat and induces the sensation of thirst, which is a powerful incentive to increasing the intake of water whereby the blood is restored to its normal concentration. The mechanism for adjusting the intake and output of water is therefore usually adequate under ordinary circumstances. There are, however, some conditions which may be benefited by increasing the intake of water. Serious depletion of water alone may occur from inability to swallow water, for example, in conditions of extreme bodily weakness, or from inability to obtain water. The water content of the body is reduced both absolutely and relatively to the salt content. Thirst is the earliest symptom. The urine is diminished in amount and the urine and plasma more concentrated. Mental confusion and hallucinations may result. The treatment is simple—water only. Usually this can be given by mouth but if the patient cannot be roused to drink adequately a 5 per cent. solution of glucose can be given parenterally.

Children, being apparently less able than adults to secrete a concentrated urine, require, in proportion to their body-weight, more water than adults to secure adequate diuresis. They are consequently less able to withstand deprivation of water. The increased flow of dilute urine resulting from drinking large quantities of water is sometimes helpful in washing out the urinary passages and in allaying irritation of their surfaces. The drinking of cold water benefits fevers by keeping the mouth clean, relieving thirst, and especially by acting as an antipyretic by facilitating perspiration and loss of heat. Drinking of water or mineral waters is also credited with beneficial effects in various diseases of metabolism such as gout or chronic rheumatism, operating in these cases presumably by facilitating the excretion of some waste products.

WATER, OSMOTIC PRESSURE AND SALT ACTION

Water is quantitatively, and perhaps even functionally, the most important constituent of the body. It forms about 70 per cent. of the body weight and is divided between the cells (which contain about three-quarters of it) and the extracellular fluids, the bulk of the latter being interstitial and the remainder in the plasma. Water is ingested in foods (which may contain half their weight of water) and swallowed as liquids. The relative amounts from these two sources will obviously vary widely but they may be about equal. Consequently much more water may be excreted in the urine than that swallowed as fluids.

Water is absorbed most rapidly from the small intestine, less rapidly from the large intestine, and hardly at all from the stomach. Water is lost from the body from the lungs as water vapour, from the skin as sweat, and from the kidney as urine. The amount lost in the breath and sweat is largely dependent on the environment, its temperature and humidity. It may be half the total in temperate climates, much more in the tropics. The kidney is less directly exposed to environmental changes and this is perhaps one reason why it has acquired the chief responsibility for regulating the water and salt content of the body.

Water absorbed from the alimentary canal brings about a dilution of the blood plasma with a resulting increased secretion of watery urine (p. 24) and a restoration of the blood to its normal osmotic pressure.

Osmotic pressure

For observing the osmotic action of salt solution on cells, the red blood corpuscles are very convenient. They are discrete cells with a definite shape and size and can be easily obtained in ample amounts. For a consideration of mere salt action, apart from the specific effect of either ion, sodium chloride is an obvious choice. It is the salt mainly responsible for the osmotic pressure of the plasma. It has another advantage that the red cells are freely permeable to water but not to sodium chloride.

If red blood corpuscles are placed in a solution of 0·9 per cent. NaCl (the concentration in which it occurs in blood plasma) they will undergo no change in size or shape. The osmotic pressure inside and outside the cell's membrane is the same and such a solution is called isotonic. If the concentration of NaCl is less (hypotonic), the cells will swell from absorption of water, and if it is sufficiently low the cells will rupture and then haemoglobin will be discharged into the fluid (haemolysis). If the concentration of NaCl be higher than 0·9 per cent. (hypertonic), water will pass out of the corpuscles into the surrounding fluid and the cells will shrink. Similar qualitative changes will occur in most cells of the body according to the variations in osmotic pressure of the extracellular fluid.

Sodium chloride

Sodium chloride is taken in the food in amounts varying perhaps from 3 to 10 G. (50 to 150 gr.) per day, and a corresponding amount is excreted daily, mainly in the urine. It is present in large and almost constant amounts in the blood and tissues. For practical purposes it may, therefore, be taken as an 'indifferent' salt, of which neither ion exerts any pronounced physiological action. Sodium chloride will, however, according to its concentration, influence the passage of fluids into or out of the cells. For maintaining the osmotic pressure of the body fluids it is the paramount constituent. Normally there is ample sodium chloride in the food for this purpose. The mechanism for maintaining osmotic pressure constant is considered later.

If a concentrated (hypertonic) solution of salt be swallowed, it will draw water from the cells of the mucous membrane of the stomach. If the quantity be small, it will be rapidly diluted, so that the effect will be transient. If the quantity be considerable, e.g. 8 G., and highly concentrated, this withdrawal of water may so irritate the cells of the mucous membrane as to set up reflex vomiting. Indeed, sodium chloride is sometimes so used as a domestic emetic.

If it reaches the intestine in concentrated solution, it will again withdraw water from the mucous membrane of the gut and so increase the amount of fluid in the intestine. In the case of sodium chloride, however, this effect will only occur in the upper part of the alimentary canal, as the salt is rapidly absorbed, so that this salt is not a saline purgative (p. 44).

Depletion of salt is being increasingly recognized as an important pathological condition. This may occur from profuse and prolonged sweating, e.g. in miners or stokers. Large amounts of both water and salts may be lost in the sweat. The primary change is decrease in the total salt content of the body. Vomiting causes a loss especially of chlorine ions, and diarrhoea of sodium ions, so that a heavy loss of both sodium chloride and water occurs in gastro-enteritis. Decreased volume of the plasma results, leading to a type of 'shock', but thirst is not a constant symptom because the concentration of the plasma is not necessarily increased. Among the symptoms are giddiness, lassitude, and painful cramps in the muscles. These are relieved by drinking salted water, water alone being ineffective. Indeed the symptoms of salt depletion due to copious sweating, where water is lost to a greater extent than salt, may only arise when thirst is satisfied by water without added salt.

OSMOTIC PRESSURE OF THE BLOOD PLASMA

So far no detailed consideration has been given to the intrinsic mechanisms whereby the osmotic pressure of the plasma is kept constant. This is largely a question of the relative amounts of water absorbed and excreted. It is closely related to another factor which admits of only limited variation—the volume of the blood which must be at least sufficient to fill the vessels so that the circulation of the blood can take place and the extravascular fluid reach all the cells of the body. The specific effect of certain ions will be discussed in the next chapter, as also the mechanism for keeping constant the reaction of the blood. All these factors are interrelated and can only be artificially separated for convenience of discussion. A brief description of the mechanism of urinary secretion will help to explain how the osmotic pressure of the plasma is regulated and will also serve as a framework for discussing the action of diuretics.

THE SECRETION OF URINE

(a) Filtration through the glomeruli

As the blood passes through the glomeruli of the kidney, water and some salts and waste products are filtered through. The amount of fluid filtered in a given time depends upon several factors: the osmotic pressure of the plasma, the pressure in the glomerular capillaries, and the rate of flow through them and their permeability. In addition to these factors which affect each individual glomerulus, the number of glomeruli functioning at a given time varies. When business is slack, some of them close down; they seem to have invented a system of 'staggered holidays'. As a result of this process a very large amount of water and solutes are filtered through the glomeruli.

(b) Reabsorption through the tubules

As the glomerular fluid passes through the kidney tubules the bulk of the water and sodium chloride and all the glucose is reabsorbed into the blood. The final volume of urine that escapes down the ureter into the bladder is, therefore, the amount excreted through the glomeruli, less the amount reabsorbed in the tubules. Diuresis depends upon the varied activities of (a) and (b), and diuretics, substances which increase the amount of urine, act by influencing one or more of these factors.

While the amount of urine depends upon the varied activities of (a) and (b), the *regulation* of the water and salt finally excreted depends mainly on reabsorption. This regulation is a function of a hormone called the *antidiuretic hormone* secreted by the posterior part of the pituitary gland and normally discharged in regular small amounts into the blood. This hormone stimulates the kidney tubules to reabsorb water and so lessens the volume of urine finally excreted. To know just when it was advisable to increase or decrease the discharge of this hormone into the blood would demand a high degree of intelligence on the part of this busy gland. It has been suggested that certain receptors in the vascular bed of the internal carotid artery are sensitive to changes in the osmotic pressure of the plasma and that nervous impulses from these 'osmoreceptors' pass through the hypothalamus, via the autonomic system, to the pituitary gland, controlling the discharge of the antidiuretic hormone, upon which therefore rests the main responsibility for keeping constant the osmotic pressure of the plasma.

The degree to which the antidiuretic hormone influences the volume of urine can be conspicuously seen from the effects of its absence in the blood. Lesions of the hypothalamic nucleus or of the posterior lobe of the pituitary gland itself can cause the condition of *diabetes insipidus*, due to imperfect reabsorption of water in the kidney tubules. There is an excessive secretion of urine (often 20 pints in 24 hours). The urine is of very low specific gravity and free from glucose (in contrast to diabetes mellitus). This necessitates the compensatory drinking of large amounts of water, to relieve thirst and avoid dehydration. This hormone has not been isolated but is associated with vaso-pressin (p. 180). The polyurea can be relieved by giving injection of vasopressin. The effect is only temporary, lasting 6–12 hours. Preparations can be given intranasally as the hormone is effec-tively absorbed from the nasal mucous membrane. The anti-diuretic hormone is released by nicotine and acetylcholine from their action on the nucleus in the hypothalamus.

DIURETICS

WATER. Water drunk by a healthy person will give a corre-sponding increase of water in the urine; to that extent water can be regarded as a diuretic. The most important therapeutic use of diuretics is, however, to get rid of excess of water from the body, and water cannot achieve this.

SALINE DIURETICS. Intake of sodium chloride, which is rapidly absorbed from the small intestine, is countered by a rapid excretion. The dissolved salt exerts a degree of osmotic pressure on the glomerular filtrate which resists absorption of water from the tubules and so increases the volume of urine. Salts which are readily absorbed and excreted can thus act as diuretics. This effect will be more pronounced if the salt has a 'low threshold' of reabsorption. Thus potassium ions have a greater diuretic action than sodium ions and nitrate ions than chloride. *Potassium Nitrate*, B.P., 0·3–1 G. (5–15 gr.), is there-fore one of the most effective saline diuretics. *Potassium Citrate*, B.P., 1–2 G. (15–30 gr.) and potassium acetate act similarly.

Alkalizing salts like sodium bicarbonate and acidifying salts like ammonium chloride (Chap. III) can also act as diuretics.

Urea, B.P. 5–15 G., U.S.P. 8–40 Gm., a low-threshold constituent of the glomerular fluid acts in the same way as salines, as a diuretic, but is used chiefly as a test for renal function (p. 314).

MERCURIAL DIURETICS

Calomel (p. 61) has long been used as a diuretic, but certain organic compounds of mercury are more powerful diuretics. Of such compounds *Mersalyl* has been much used. It contains about 40 per cent. of mercury in a non-ionizable form, and is administered parenterally as a specially prepared injection, *Injection of Mersalyl*, B.P., *Mersalyl and Theophylline Injection*, U.S.P. This injection contains 10 per cent. of mersalyl and 5 per cent. theophylline, the addition of theophylline, which is itself a diuretic, preventing the decomposition, with consequent increased toxicity, of the mercurial compound. It is usual to begin with a small dose, perhaps 0·5 ml. by deep intramuscular injection, with subsequent injections of doses up to 2 ml. at intervals of two or more days, as conditions determine. Only if the response to intramuscular injection is unsatisfactory should the injection be given intravenously. In cases of oedema due to congestive heart failure, mersalyl may produce an enormous diuresis, amounting to 3 to 5 litres in 24 hours. The diuretic effect may be increased by previous administration of ammonium chloride or nitrate for a few days, but this is usually unnecessary.

Meralluride, *Mercurophylline*, and *Sterile Mercaptomerin Sodium* are other organic mercurials, prepared as *Injections* for use as diuretics. Mercurophylline may also be given by mouth.

All these substances act by diminishing reabsorption from the tubules, by formation of mercaptides which effect the removal of labile —SH groups from those enzymes in the renal tubules which are necessary for reabsorption of Cl^-.

XANTHINE COMPOUNDS. *Caffeine*, *Theobromine*, and *Theo-*

phylline are important diuretics but for convenience of consideration of their other actions they are discussed later (p. 78).

PLASMA SUBSTITUTES

In certain cases of severe dehydration it may be urgently necessary to restore the blood volume. For reasons previously explained a solution used for intravenous injection would have to be isotonic with the plasma. 'Normal Saline' solution containing 0·9 per cent. of sodium chloride, *Injection of Sodium Chloride*, B.P., U.S.P., would satisfy this requirement. *Compound Injection of Sodium Chloride*, B.P., *Ringer's Injection*, U.S.P., would be preferable in so far as it is not only correct osmotically but also supplies the plasma with the salts, Na, K, and Ca, in the proportions in which they occur in the plasma itself. It was found, however, that these solutions are of little value because if injected intravenously they pass so rapidly into the tissues and urine that only a transient increase in blood volume occurs and oedema may be produced.

Human blood plasma or serum is much more effective, as the colloids serve to retain the water in the blood. They have been widely used in cases of plasma loss due to burns.

Official in the B.P. are *Liquid Human Serum* (*Normal Human Serum Albumin*, U.S.P.) and *Dried Human Serum* (which is easier to transport and keeps longer and is reconstituted by the addition of sterile saline solution) and *Dried Human Plasma* (*Normal Human Plasma*, U.S.P.).

The difficulty of obtaining sufficient amounts of human plasma has stimulated the search for substances which, in appropriate solution, could act as substitutes for plasma. Such a solution should possess the following properties: its osmotic pressure and viscosity should approximate closely to those of blood; the molecules should be of such a size that they will not leave the vessels too freely but eventual elimination must be complete; the substance must be non-toxic and non-antigenic. These conditions are not too easy to satisfy. Of such substances, *Dextran*, a polysaccharide, has been widely used.

BLOOD TRANSFUSION

In cases where a dangerous diminution in the red cells has occurred, e.g. after severe haemorrhage, nothing but *transfusion of blood* itself may be of any avail. This not only supplies a fluid of the right osmotic pressure and viscosity, but restores the oxygen-carrying capacity of the blood. Naturally, the technique of blood transfusion is much more complicated than that of intravenous injection of saline solutions, and, for supplying the blood, a donor must be found whose red cells have no toxic (agglutinative or haemolytic) action on the blood of the patient.

For this purpose the B.P. and the U.S.P. provide *Whole Human Blood,* which is extensively used, after due precautions about compatibility, in replacement of blood loss. Occasionally special cases need a replacement of red corpuscles rather than of total blood volume (aplastic and other anaemias) and use may be made of *Concentrated Human Red Blood Corpuscles.* Other preparations of the globulin fractions of plasma protein are in use for the immunity to acquired disease which they confer.

III

KATIONS OF THE BLOOD: ACIDS AND ALKALIS

INTRODUCTION

ABOUT a century ago, Claude Bernard pointed out that, for the normal functioning of the cells of the body, they had to be surrounded by a fluid of particular composition, which could only be varied within very narrow limits—the *Milieu Intérieur*. It is a remarkable fact that the ratios of Na, K, and Ca in the plasma are almost constant throughout the vertebrate kingdom and that these ratios closely resemble the ratios in sea-water. The suggestion has been made that the ionic content of the blood dates back to that of the sea from which living organisms first emerged. That, starting from a single-celled organism in the sea, a mammal, living on land with all its environmental changes, can still contrive that its cells should live in an environment so similar, in regard to salt content, to the sea, is an astounding feat. Fortunately evolution was in no pressing hurry. It took millions of years.

Ringer found that, while a frog's heart would beat for some time in a solution of sodium chloride, isotonic with frog's plasma, it would beat much longer and more efficiently if the fluid contained also calcium and potassium in suitable concentrations, calcium facilitating contraction of the heart and potassium relaxation. Ringer established the composition of such a solution suitable for frog's tissues (Ringer's Solution) and corresponding solutions (e.g. Locke's Solution) were afterwards determined for mammalian tissues. Subsequent work has established the importance of such a balanced solution for the proper functioning of all tissues. In the previous chapter the salts of the plasma have been considered mainly from the point of view of their osmotic properties. Since Ringer's classical experiments, it has become increasingly evident that, both for normal function and in pathological conditions, the kations of the blood have important individual actions beyond their mere osmotic effects. These will now be dealt with.

SODIUM

The sodium ion may be regarded as possessing no specific physiological action. Sodium chloride is present in so many foodstuffs and the body mechanisms are so adapted to conserve it that only under exceptional conditions (p. 22) can any serious *depletion* occur.

Hormones play an important part in the regulation of sodium and potassium and, in deficiency of these hormones (e.g. Addison's disease), there is an increased loss of sodium and a retention of potassium (p. 219).

SODIUM RETENTION. In some pathological conditions the body cannot excrete sufficient sodium to maintain a proper balance. This sodium holds back water and lessens its excretion. Oedema may result. This is liable to occur in congestive heart failure, when the kidney cannot excrete sufficient sodium, possibly due to low glomerular filtration, secondary to reduced renal blood flow. In these conditions oedema may be greatly reduced by a *low salt diet*, with which it is unnecessary to reduce the intake of fluids.

POTASSIUM

The potassium ion is essential for functionally balanced body fluids or for physiological solutions like Ringer's solution. Normally there is an ample supply of potassium in the diet to maintain the body requirements, and excretion by the kidney is so rapid as to prevent any of the toxic effects that an excess of potassium may produce. Potassium salts, when *injected intravenously* in sufficient amounts, depress the activity of muscular tissues, especially of the heart. No such results normally follow the *oral ingestion* of potassium salts. In nephritis, where the excretion of potassium is unduly diminished, even the oral administration of potassium salts may lead to a sufficient rise in the blood concentration to cause some cardiac depression, and in Addison's disease symptoms may be partly due to potassium retention. Ordinarily, however, there is no significant difference between the actions of a sodium salt and the corresponding potassium salt except that the diuretic action of the latter may be greater.

POTASSIUM DEPLETION. This has received increasing recognition in recent years, starting from recognition of its occurrence in infantile gastro-enteritis. The condition is less easy to demonstrate than sodium depletion, because potassium is an electrolyte mainly of intracellular fluid, but it is possibly at least as common. The renal defence of body potassium is relatively inefficient, in that it is excreted even on a low potassium diet, in contrast to the retention of sodium on a low sodium diet. Even so, potassium is so widely distributed in foods that depletion is very unlikely to arise from dietetic errors. It has been recognized in patients with severe diarrhoea and vomiting, during the recovery phase of diabetic coma, during convalescence from surgical operations, and from overdosage with adrenocortical hormones. Paresis of muscles and generalized weakness are the outstanding clinical effects of lowered extracellular potassium concentration. Potassium facilitates the passage of impulses from motor nerves to voluntary muscles. In a rare disease, familial periodic paralysis, the administration of large doses of potassium chloride may so improve conduction as to avert or abolish the symptoms of paralysis. A less striking relief of paretic symptoms may result in myasthenia gravis (p. 147) from giving potassium salts.

To correct depletion, *Potassium Chloride* may be given by mouth or, in urgent cases, intravenously. The latter method is not without risk and the solution should not exceed 0·5 per cent. potassium and must be injected slowly.

CALCIUM

Calcium to the amount of about 10 mg. in 100 ml. is normally and constantly present in the blood. Ringer showed that calcium is necessary for a balanced physiological solution, e.g. for maintaining the beat of the perfused heart. It is now known to be equally necessary for the functional activity of nearly all tissues. A normal diet sufficiently provides for the calcium requirements of the body and for the replacement of the continual loss by excretion through the kidneys and bowel. It is mainly by the selective excretion through these organs, together with the action of parathyroid hormone (p. 216), that the calcium in the blood is kept constant in spite of variations of intake. Vitamin D (p. 235) increases the absorption of calcium.

No condition is known in which there is any advantage in raising the calcium content of the tissues above the normal. From the limited point of view of therapeutics, therefore, calcium is used only in conditions in which the supply of it to the tissues is defective.

In childhood the rapid growth of bones makes unusual demands on calcium, and similarly, during pregnancy, the foetal requirements must be met indirectly through the food of the mother. In those cases it is important that the supply of calcium in the diet, never greatly in excess of the requirements, should be abundant. Milk is one of the best sources of calcium in the diet.

Apart from these physiological conditions, there are certain diseases associated with deranged calcium metabolism. In rickets the softness of the bones is due mainly to defective calcium deposition, but the error does not lie so much in deficiency of calcium as of Vitamin D in the food, and lime salts have, *per se*, little or no beneficial action.

One result of serious deficiency of lime salts in the tissues is an increased excitability of the neuromuscular system which may lead to 'tetany' (contractions of certain groups of muscles) or even more generalized convulsions. This may occur in rickets, and requires treatment by Vitamin D and lime salts.

An ionized calcium salt is necessary for coagulation of the

blood, taking part in the conversion of prothrombin into thrombin. Bleeding diseases are rarely, if ever, due to low calcium content of the blood, and consequently calcium therapy is usually valueless (p. 207).

Calcium salts have an action in diminishing the permeability of animal membranes. In diseases such as urticaria, serum rash, and chilblains, where there is undue permeability of the capillaries, calcium salts are sometimes beneficial. Parathyroid extract can also increase the blood calcium (p. 216).

Calcium salts given by mouth are largely converted into insoluble carbonates which diminishes their absorption; after absorption they are excreted partly by the intestinal mucous membrane as carbonates. One result of this is that the administration of chloride of calcium has the effect of diminishing the alkali reserve of the blood. Whether the calcium of calcium chloride is retained or excreted in the intestine as carbonate, the result is to free chloride in the body which then combines with and diminishes the reserve alkali forming sodium chloride. As more of the sodium base is thus excreted as neutral chloride, there is less available to combine with phosphates, and consequently the ratio of acid phosphate is increased in the urine and the urine rendered more acid. The amount of urine is also increased.

When an increase in the absorption of calcium is desired, soluble salts must be given. In chronic conditions they may be given by mouth, with addition of Vitamin D in appropriate cases. *Calcium Lactate*, B.P., 1–4 G. (15–60 gr.), is a suitable salt as it does not affect the alkaline reserve like the chloride, and is also less irritant than the latter. *Calcium Gluconate*, B.P., 1–4 G. (15–60 gr.), U.S.P., 5 Gm., has also been widely used and can be given by mouth or by intramuscular or intravenous injection (*Injection of Calcium Gluconate*, B.P., 10–20 ml. (1–2 G.), U.S.P., 1 Gm.).

Calcium Carbonate, B.P., an insoluble salt, has long been used in the form of prepared chalk as a remedy for diarrhoea. Especially in acid diarrhoeas in children, it probably acts mainly as an antacid, but it may also diminish the permeability of the mucous membrane of the gut, and thus restrain the excessive passage of fluid into the lumen of the intestine. *Chalk*, B.P., is given in doses of 1–4 G. (15–60 gr.). It can be conveniently prescribed in the form of *Aromatic Powder of Chalk*, B.P., dose 0·6–4 G. (10–60 gr.). The U.S.P. has *Precipitated Calcium Carbonate*, 1 Gm.

AMMONIUM

Ammonium is present in the blood only in small amounts and does not possess the physiological importance of sodium, potassium, or calcium. The uncomplicated action of the ammonium ion is naturally displayed most simply by *Ammonium Chloride*, B.P., U.S.P. This neutral salt is freely soluble and, as the ammonium is combined with a strong acid, the salt is relatively stable and does not smell of ammonia. Given by mouth, ammonium chloride, though it is rapidly absorbed, produces no specific effects of the ammonium ion, because, like potassium chloride, it is so rapidly excreted. If injected intravenously it stimulates the central nervous system, but is not used therapeutically for this.

Large doses of ammonium chloride given by mouth cause a reduction of the alkaline reserve of the blood, as it is converted by the liver into urea and hydrochloric acid. This reduction of reserve alkali increases the amount of urine and renders it more acid. Ammonium chloride is given for this purpose in a divided daily dose of 4 G.

Ammonium Bicarbonate, B.P., *Ammonium Carbonate*, U.S.P. (a mixture of bicarbonate and carbamate), in contradistinction to ammonium chloride, is unstable and decomposes rapidly with the liberation of ammonia. Owing to its alkalinity and its liberating NH_3, it is used rather for local actions than for the effect of the ammonium ion after absorption.

In the stomach, ammonium carbonate acts as a local antacid and irritates the mucous membrane. It reflexly increases the bronchial secretion like other gastric irritants, and is sometimes used as an expectorant in doses of 0·3 G. (5 gr.). Larger doses 0·6–2 G. (10–30 gr.) produce emesis. As it is rapidly converted into urea by the liver, ammonium carbonate does not increase the alkalinity of the urine.

The gas NH_3 comes off readily from ammonium carbonate or hydrate. When inhaled, it irritates the nasal mucous membrane. This irritation produces reflex stimulation of the medullary centres. Ammonium carbonate is thus often used in the form of smelling-salts to stimulate those centres in cases of fainting or collapse.

When a solution of ammonium carbonate is swallowed, similar reflex effects occur from irritation of the mouth and upper part of the alimentary canal. *Aromatic Ammonia Spirit*, U.S.P., 2 ml., which contains ammonia, ammonium carbonate, and certain volatile oils in alcohol, is a favourite preparation for internal administration. The B.P. has now replaced the carbonate by the bicarbonate, which is of more constant composition but similar in action. The B.P. *Aromatic Spirit of Ammonia*, 1–4 ml. (15–60 min.), is similar in composition to the U.S.P. spirit.

MAGNESIUM

Magnesium is slowly absorbed (like calcium) and rapidly excreted. In the presence of normal kidney function it is therefore unusual for any excess to occur. In the body, most of it is found within the cells although some is present in serum in ionized form. When injected, magnesium salts depress the nervous system. Locally they may cause loss of sensation. A fall of blood pressure occurs after intravenous administration from blocking of conduction in the sympathetic ganglia and depression of the brain may cause loss of consciousness. Peripherally the conduction of impulses from the motor nerves to the skeletal muscle fibres is also depressed, which may produce a flaccid paralysis. Little use is made of these actions in therapeutics.

The difficulty of absorption permits of the use of salts of magnesium for their local actions, e.g. *Magnesium Sulphate* as a saline purgative (p. 44) or to withdraw pus and infected material from abscess cavities when applied externally as a compress (magnesium sulphate paste). These actions are due to the osmotic activity of the soluble but unabsorbed salt. In addition use is made of *Magnesium Oxide* (p. 39) as an antacid.

ACIDS AND ALKALIS

REACTION OF THE BLOOD. In Chapter II consideration was given to the mechanisms whereby the osmotic pressure of the plasma is kept constant and to the methods which can be used to correct pathological deviations from normal osmotic pressure. Another property of the blood, of at least equal importance, is its reaction, which admits of variation only within very narrow limits. Life is in fact possible only when the reaction of the body fluids is slightly on the alkaline side of neutrality. The devices which the body uses to attain this essential end are complicated but a brief account may be given of the chief methods by which the acid-base balance is maintained.

In the blood there are fixed kations (Na^+, &c.) combined with fixed anions (e.g. Cl^-) and with labile anions (e.g. HCO_3^-). During exercise (liberation of lactic acid), in disease (acidosis) or after administration of acid salts, excess of fixed acid is formed in the blood. This fixed acid is neutralized chiefly by the sodium bicarbonate which forms the normal alkali reserve of the body fluids. The displaced CO_2 stimulates the respiratory centre and is eliminated by the augmented respiration. This restores the *reaction* of the blood, but at the expense of the alkali reserve, which depends mainly on the total available amount of sodium bicarbonate, some of which has been removed in the process. The diminished alkaline reserve is countered by the excretion of fixed acid salts in the urine. The ratio of acid phosphate to alkaline phosphate in the urine is increased, and the urine becomes more acid. Thus a compensated acidosis merely alters the alkali reserve of the blood and not the true blood pH. Should the latter occur from failure of these mechanisms, death would follow.

When the body has to cope with an increase in the alkali of

the blood, e.g. after administration of sodium bicarbonate, a converse process occurs. The base absorbed from the small intestine increases the amount of alkali in the body (the alkali reserve) but again there is little or no change in the pH of the blood because an increased amount of base is excreted in the urine making it less acid as well as increasing its amount. When excessive amounts of alkaline salts are absorbed, the alkali reserve rises and there is a diminution of chlorides in the blood and urine. Toxic symptoms may occur, including vomiting, mental impairment, and tetany.

ACIDS

Some acids owe their physiological action almost entirely to their acidity, i.e. to the hydrogen ion, and these may be taken together here. In the case of other acids like hydrocyanic acid, the negative ion is so toxic that the part played by acidity is negligible. As the degree of acidity depends upon the amount of dissociation of the acid, the effects to be described will of course vary with the solubility and degree of dissociation. In the case of salicylic acid, which is only slightly soluble and feebly dissociated, the acid action is of relatively little importance.

Strong acids exert a powerful caustic action, due chiefly to their neutralizing alkalis and precipitating some of the proteins. They cause blistering and destruction of the skin, and mucous membranes are even more sensitive to their corrosive action. When swallowed, such acids produce the typical symptoms of corrosive poisoning; pain in the mouth and stomach, vomiting, and collapse.

Dilute acids have a characteristic taste, and induce a reflex flow of saliva. Solutions of citric acid or preparations of lemon, which have a pleasant taste and relieve thirst, are used to make a cooling drink in fevers.

Pure gastric juice is normally acid and contains about 0·5 per cent. of hydrochloric acid. The acidity of the stomach contents during digestion of a mixed meal is usually about half that concentration. This acid is necessary for activation of pepsin. No advantage is gained by increasing the gastric acid above the normal, but in achlorhydria and other diseases where this acid is deficient or absent (e.g. in pernicious anaemia) this defect can to some extent be made good and digestion improved by administration of dilute hydrochloric acid, though it is practically impossible to give enough acid completely to replace the amount secreted. For internal administration **Dilute Hydrochloric Acid**, B.P., 0·6–8 ml. (10–120 min.) 10 per cent. solution, is given well diluted.

Acids are usually absorbed rapidly from the alimentary canal, but do not exist in the blood or tissues as acids as they are neutralized chiefly by the alkaline bicarbonate of the blood. On account of their local and other actions, mineral acids are not used therapeutically for their actions after absorption and cannot conveniently be given in amounts sufficient to produce any marked or lasting effect on the reaction of the urine.

The *Acidity of the Urine* may with advantage be increased in certain conditions. It has been shown that any excess of fixed acid in the blood is countered partly by excretion of NaH_2PO_4 in the urine. This salt, **Sodium Acid Phosphate**, B.P., given by mouth is excreted as such in the urine and can be used to increase its acidity in a daily divided dose of 4 G.

As increase of acidity checks the growth of some microorganisms, acid sodium phosphate may also act as a urinary antiseptic. Any considerable increase in the acidity of the urine cannot, however, be kept up for long, owing to the irritation of the urinary passages which it produces. In the U.S.P. this salt is called **Sodium Biphosphate** (600 mg.–1 Gm.).

Calcium Chloride (p. 33) and **Ammonium Chloride** (p. 34) may also be used to make the urine more acid. They are more effective than sodium acid phosphate and are now usually preferred to it.

ALKALIS

In the case of the hydrates and carbonate of sodium and potassium, the action of the metal is negligible compared with

that of the —OH ion, so that the action of these compounds
may be regarded as due entirely to their alkalinity. The hydrates,
being more freely dissociated, are more energetic in action than
the carbonates or bicarbonates.

Strong alkalis, especially the *hydrates* like caustic potash,
are powerful corrosives, chiefly owing to their dissolving proteins and neutralizing acids, and will thus produce destruction
and necrosis of tissues with which they come in contact. Solutions of the *carbonates*, while less caustic, can also produce
much irritation, especially if they are allowed prolonged action.
The ingestion of poisonous amounts of alkalis, especially in
concentrated solution, causes corrosion of the mouth, oesophagus, and stomach. Death may occur from perforation of the
stomach or shock. If the corrosion is not so severe and the
patient recovers from the shock and collapse, gastric ulcer or
cicatrices may occur. Apart from this caustic action, the alkalis,
like acids, are of importance chiefly from the effects they produce on the alimentary canal, blood, and urine.

GASTRIC ANTACIDS. In cases of hyperacidity of the stomach,
alkalis, by neutralizing the excess of acid, relieve the pain and
eructation. A carbonate is less suitable for this purpose, because the carbonic acid liberated seems to stimulate gastric
secretion and therefore to increase the acidity after a temporary
diminution. For this purpose, therefore, a carbonate like
Sodium Bicarbonate, though widely used as an antacid, is inferior to an oxide like magnesium oxide. Weight for weight, the
latter can neutralize four times as much acid as can sodium
bicarbonate. Calcium carbonate (p. 33) and bismuth carbonate
(p. 68) are also used as stomach antacids though the latter has
a very feeble neutralizing action.

Insoluble itself, *Magnesium Oxide* (Magnesia) combines
with hydrochloric acid in the stomach to form the soluble
magnesium chloride. It therefore not only acts as an antacid
(0·3 G. (5 gr.) repeated) but will purge, like magnesium sulphate, if given in sufficient doses, 2–4 G. (30–60 gr.). Magnesium
oxide tends to purge, while calcium and bismuth carbonates

have the opposite effect. By a judicious combination of these three, hyperchlorhydria can be reduced with but little interference with the intestinal functions. Combinations of these three are frequently used in the treatment of gastric ulcers.

Magnesium Trisilicate, B.P. 0·3–2 G. (5–30 gr.), U.S.P. 1 Gm., is much favoured to lessen acidity of the stomach. It acts largely by adsorption of the acid which is subsequently released and neutralized in the intestine, and has a soothing effect in indigestion by lining inflamed areas of the mucosa with a gelatinous protective layer. For this reason in addition to their properties of adsorbing and neutralizing acid, *Aluminum Hydroxide* and *Phosphate Gels*, U.S.P., are also widely used, either as fluid suspensions or tablets, flavoured with the carminative peppermint oil.

Overdosage with a soluble alkali like sodium bicarbonate may produce serious alkalosis with tetany; this does not occur with adsorbents like magnesium trisilicate or aluminium hydroxide, which can be given for long periods without producing toxic effects.

A reduction of the alkaline reserve of the blood (acidosis) occurs in a variety of diseases, including uraemia, diabetes, and shock. In these conditions sodium bicarbonate may produce a temporary improvement. It may be given by mouth, 1–2 G. (15–30 gr.) or intravenously as 5 per cent. *Injection of Sodium Bicarbonate*, B.P.,

Alkalis are frequently prescribed in order to lessen the acidity of the urine, especially when this is giving rise to irritation or pain in the urinary passages. For this purpose sodium or potassium bicarbonate can be given (20–30 gr. or more) as they are excreted by the urine as carbonates and so diminish its acidity. They also from their salt action (p. 21) increase the secretion of urine.

Acetates or *Citrates* of *Sodium* or *Potassium* have actions on the blood and urine similar to those of bicarbonates, because the citrates and acetates are oxidized in the tissues to carbonates and bicarbonates, and are excreted as such. They have the advantage over the carbonates in interfering less with digestion, as they do not so much reduce the acidity of the stomach contents. They are given as alkaline diuretics in doses of 1–4 G. (15–60 gr.). *Potassium* and *Sodium Citrates* are official in the B.P. and Sodium Citrate in the U.S.P.

Citrates form unionized, though soluble, salts with calcium and so prevent coagulation of the blood. Sodium citrate is used for this purpose, e.g. when blood, or plasma is collected for transfusion. For this and similar purposes, there are available *Anticoagulant Sodium Citrate Solution*, U.S.P., and a similar solution containing dextrose.

IV

DRUGS ACTING ON THE ALIMENTARY CANAL

As drugs are in the majority of cases given by mouth, they naturally have every opportunity of exerting any local action they may have on the mucous membrane of the alimentary canal as they pass through. Also the glands and muscle of the alimentary canal can be influenced in a variety of ways—directly, reflexly, or through their nervous system. Consequently, a very large number of drugs have some action on the alimentary canal. Those to be considered here are such as owe their chief medicinal importance to this action. Other drugs, belonging to such different groups as, for example, atropine, carbachol, and mercury, have important actions on the alimentary canal, but with these drugs the action on the digestive tube is rather an incident in a wider sphere of action for which they may be more conveniently considered elsewhere.

DRUGS ACTING ON THE STOMACH

SIMPLE BITTERS. This group includes a number of drugs which have little in common beyond their bitter taste and absence of physiological action. They are used to improve appetite and to stimulate gastric secretions. This they do reflexly through the sense of taste and most effectively if given shortly before meals. Any substance possessing a bitter taste will do this. Nearly all alkaloids are bitter, but they usually have more important actions. Simple bitters have little action, in medicinal doses, apart from this effect on digestion due to their bitter taste.

Of the many vegetable substances which have been used as bitters, Gentian is now the most commonly employed. One favourite preparation of it is *Compound Tincture of Gentian,*

B.P., which is made from gentian, orange peel, and cardamoms, and has an agreeable aromatic bitter taste. It is given in doses of 2–4 ml. (30–60 min.) and much used in mixtures.

ACIDS. When gastric digestion is deranged from lack of hydrochloric acid (achlorhydria) as, for example, in pernicious anaemia and in carcinoma of the stomach, dilute hydrochloric acid may be given with benefit (p. 38). The official *Dilute Hydrochloric Acid*, B.P., contains 10 per cent. of hydrochloric acid and is given in doses of 0·6–8 ml. (10–120 min.), well diluted.

ALKALIS. In cases where the stomach secretes too much acid (hyperchlorhydria) alkalis can be given to neutralize the excess of acid (p. 39) and are sometimes called gastric antacids.

CARMINATIVES. Certain aromatic and volatile substances have been found to aid in the expulsion, by eructation, of gas accumulated in the stomach. This they do apparently by relaxing the cardiac orifice. They thus frequently relieve discomfort due to distension of the stomach. Among the substances used for this action ('carminative' action) may be mentioned volatile oils, e.g. of peppermint, and other volatile substances such as alcohol, chloroform water, &c. Sodium Bicarbonate, by liberating CO_2 in the stomach, may also exert a carminative action.

DRUGS ACTING ON THE INTESTINE: PURGATIVES

Generally speaking, purgatives act either by making the contents of the intestine more fluid or by rendering the movements of the intestine more active, or by a combination of these actions. Such effects can be produced in a variety of ways in accordance with which purgatives can roughly be classified.

The chief normal stimulus to peristaltic activity is the bulk of the intestinal contents, which depends largely upon the amount of unabsorbable material in the food. The latter can be increased artificially by giving with the food some indifferent unabsorbable material. *Agar*, U.S.P., a preparation made from seaweed and consisting largely of unabsorbable gelose which forms a jelly with water, is sometimes given for this purpose. It not only adds to the bulk of the contents of the bowel but also retains water and prevents its absorption. It thus acts as a gentle laxative. It is almost tasteless and is given in doses of 4 Gm., with food or in water.

Liquid Paraffin, B.P., *Liquid Petrolatum*, U.S.P., achieves the same purpose in a different way. It is a mixture of liquid hydrocarbons obtained from petroleum and is a tasteless fluid of oily consistency, which is non-irritant and is not absorbed from the intestine. It is given in doses of 8–30 ml. ($\frac{1}{4}$–1 fl. oz.). This adds something to the bulk of the intestinal contents but especially acts as a lubricant. It has been much used in the treatment of chronic constipation.

SALINE PURGATIVES

Ions differ greatly in the readiness with which they are absorbed from the alimentary canal. The chief action of 'diffusible' salts—i.e. salts which are readily absorbed—in medicinal doses is the diuretic action (p. 25). But salts which are 'indiffusible' cannot, when given by mouth, exert this diuretic action, which is dependent upon their being absorbed. If given in sufficient quantity, indiffusible salts act as purgatives. Again, only such salts will be useful for this purpose if their ions have otherwise no pronounced actions which would prevent the salts being given in considerable amounts. It has been found that of such salts, the kation Mg and the sulphate, phosphate, and tartrate anions are especially indiffusible. Diffusibility must not be confused with solubility; actually magnesium sulphate, though indiffusible, is extremely soluble.

Injected into a ligatured loop of the intestine, water itself or an isotonic solution of sodium chloride is rapidly absorbed, but an isotonic solution of *Magnesium Sulphate* is not. Magnesium sulphate will not pass easily through the mucous membrane, and water can only be absorbed from the solution to a limited extent, if any, because, as the water is absorbed and the solution therefore becomes more concentrated, greater energy is required to absorb the water against the rising osmotic pressure inside the intestine. The effect of an isotonic solution of magnesium sulphate will therefore be to retard the absorption of water. If the solution is hypotonic, some water will be absorbed from it and thereafter the result will be the same. This is one way in which salts are given as purgatives, i.e. in *isotonic* or *hypotonic solution*. The bulk of the intestinal contents is increased and rendered more fluid by the amount of solution given. The increase in the bulk incites reflex peristalsis, and the increased fluidity facilitates the passage of the intestinal contents. A 6 per cent. solution of magnesium sulphate is about isotonic with the body fluids, and therefore a dose of 6 G. (90 gr.) will retain about 100 ml. of water in the gut. A dose of 90 gr. dissolved in 100 ml. or more of water is a usual dose for this action of retarding the absorption of water. Purgation usually results in from 1 to 3 hours.

If a *hypertonic solution* of magnesium sulphate be placed inside a ligatured loop of the intestine, it will draw water from the mucous membrane into the lumen, in addition to preventing absorption of the water in which it is itself dissolved. A given dose of magnesium sulphate may, perhaps contrary to expectation, act more slowly as a purgative in hypertonic than in isotonic solution. This is because it will take some time for the former to withdraw water so as to give a bulk of fluid equal to that of the isotonic solution and also because the hypertonic solution, by causing temporary closure of the pyloric sphincter, may delay the passage of the stomach contents into the intestine. Larger doses of magnesium sulphate, 8–16 G. (120–240 gr.) are sometimes given in hypertonic solution with the definite intention of withdrawing water from the body by way of the intestine, or for the secondary effect of diminishing the blood-volume and concentrating the blood. Such a concentrated solution of an unabsorbable salt will diminish the secretion of urine, owing to the increased concentration of the blood—an effect which may be contrasted with the diuretic effect of an easily absorbable salt like potassium citrate.

A saline purgative like magnesium sulphate increases peristalsis only indirectly as a result of the increased bulk and fluidity of the intestinal contents. More effective purgation can be produced if it be combined with a drug like senna which directly stimulates peristalsis. As saline purgatives act quickly they are usually given first thing in the morning and followed by hot tea or coffee. They are so used when a thorough and speedy evacuation is desired. Small doses taken regularly before breakfast will in many people counteract chronic constipation.

In the case of magnesium sulphate, both ions are indiffusible, but much the same effects are produced by a soluble salt only one of whose ions is indiffusible, because one ion cannot be absorbed without the other. Thus *Magnesium Chloride* and *Sodium Sulphate*, *Sodium Phosphate*, and *Potassium Sodium Tartrate* act as purgatives in the same way as magnesium sulphate.

A convenient way of administering these saline purgatives is in the form of an effervescent powder, of which Seidlitz Powder, *Compound Effervescent Powder*, B.P., may be taken as an example. This is dispensed in two packets, one in blue paper containing sodium bicarbonate and sodium potassium tartrate, the other in white paper containing tartaric acid. The first is dissolved in water and the contents of the white packet (previously dissolved by preference) are added to the solution, which is drunk during effervescence. The effervescence is of course provided by the CO_2 liberated from the sodium bicarbonate by the action of tartaric acid. The effervescence not only masks the salt taste to some extent, but is believed to make the solution act more quickly, possibly by hastening the passage from the stomach into the intestine.

When magnesium salts are given by mouth, the systemic actions of magnesium do not come into play, because the small amounts of magnesium that are absorbed are as rapidly excreted (p. 35).

Sulphur itself has no physiological activity owing to its insolubility in the body fluids. When taken internally some of it is changed into hydrogen sulphide and other sulphides. These act as mild irritants and increase peristalsis, usually with the painless passage of a soft formed stool. *Precipitated Sulphur*, B.P., U.S.P., is thus often used as a mild laxative in doses of 1–4 G. (15–60 gr.). Some of the ingested sulphur may be absorbed and excreted mainly by the skin as sulphides, and by the kidney as sulphates. It may thus act as a mild diaphoretic and diuretic, which may explain the beneficial effects resulting from sulphur medication or sulphur waters in the treatment of chronic rheumatism and chronic skin diseases. Applied to the skin in ointment, sulphur is partly changed into sulphides, which are destructive to certain animal parasites but have little action on bacteria. In skin diseases due to the former (e.g. scabies) ointment of sulphur has been much used (p. 310).

Castor Oil, B.P., is a fixed oil obtained from *Ricinus communis*, a plant native to India but cultivated in many parts of the globe. The oil was known to the Egyptians and Greeks, but fell into neglect until Dr. Cavare, a physician of Bath who had practised in the West Indies, recommended it in 1764 as a gentle purgative. Since then it has become widely used as one of the safest and mildest of purgatives.

Castor oil is a pale yellowish transparent viscid liquid, having a faint odour and a slight but nauseating taste. Like other fixed oils and fats, it is an ester of a fatty acid—in this case ricinoleic acid—with glycerol. So long as the fatty acid is combined with glycerol the oil is non-irritant, and so can be applied to the skin or even mucous membranes as an emollient. When ingested, it passes unchanged through the stomach, but in the intestine is split up, like other fats, by the fat-splitting ferment of the pancreas (lipase) into its two constituents— glycerol and ricinoleic acid. The freed fatty acid acts as a mild irritant to the gut and so provokes purgation.

It acts in from 2 to 8 hours, and produces soft but not watery motions. It is a very safe purgative and has little tendency to cause griping. Hence it can be used in cases where more violent purgatives are contra-indicated, e.g. in infants, for the aged, and during pregnancy. Its chief drawback is its slight but disagreeable taste and smell. This can be well disguised by giving it with orange juice. The dose is from 4–16 ml. (60–240 min.) for an adult. Half a teaspoonful or more can be given to an infant. Ricin, a protein which causes violent gastro-intestinal irritation when ingested and which is highly toxic when injected, is present in the castor-oil seeds but not in the oil itself.

RESINOUS PURGATIVES

Many substances containing resinous bodies as active principles, e.g. Jalap and Colocynth, have been used as purgatives but are now obsolescent. They act usually in 2–4 hours with watery stools and sometimes with colic. *Podophyllum Resin*, B.P., 15–60 mg. ($\frac{1}{4}$–1 gr.), is still in occasional use.

ANTHRACENE GROUP OF PURGATIVES

This important group of purgatives, which includes cascara, senna, aloes, and rhubarb, may be taken together, because each of them owes its action to active principles which are derivatives of anthracene ($C_{14}H_{10}$). Owing to this similarity in their active principles, they have similar pharmacological properties. They act mainly on the large intestine, stimulating the contractions of the muscle. They are slow in action, requiring 8–12 or more hours to produce purgation. It has been shown, especially in the case of senna, that the drug contains the anthracene bodies combined with sugars to form inactive glucosides. These glucosides are absorbed slowly from the small intestine and converted in the body to active compounds (e.g. emodin) which stimulate the muscle of the large bowel through the blood stream. The delay in action is, therefore, due to the time required for absorption and conversion into active compounds. As they stimulate the muscular movements, they are liable to cause griping if given alone, but this can usually be prevented by prescribing along with them something which relieves excessive intestinal contractions, e.g. a volatile oil or hyoscyamus. As constipation is frequently due to inertia of the large bowel, these purgatives are frequently used in its treatment, but they should only be used as adjuvants to the more important treatment of constipation by diet, exercise, and regular habits. Chrysophanic acid, one of the anthracene bodies found in rhubarb and senna, may cause a yellowish coloration of the urine if acid, or reddish if it is alkaline.

Cascara Sagrada, B.P., U.S.P., the dried bark of *Rhamnus purshianus*, is one of the mildest of this group, and in the treatment of chronic constipation is frequently given in small repeated doses of the *Liquid Extract of Cascara Sagrada*, B.P., or the *Elixir of Cascara Sagrada*, B.P., both 2–4 ml. (30–60 min.), or the *Aromatic Fluid extract*, U.S.P., 2 ml. The *Dry Extract of Cascar Sagrada*, B.P., 0·12–0·5 G. (2–8 gr.) is usually made into tablets.

Senna Leaf, B.P., the dried leaves of various species of Cassia, shrubs which grow in Africa, India, and elsewhere, has been used for centuries as a purgative. Senna is used in a variety of preparations. *Compound Powder of Liquorice*, B.P., 4–8 G. (60–120 gr.) owes its purgative action to the Senna and Sulphur contained in it. Liquorice, a sweet substance which gives the powder its name, serves to conceal the disagreeable taste of Senna. The powder also contains Fennel, a volatile oil which tends to prevent the griping which Senna is liable to produce.

The B.P. contains the *Senna Fruit* in addition to the leaf. From it several preparations are made including *Syrup of Senna*, B.P., 2–8 ml. (30–120 min.).

Aloes, B.P., is the dried juice obtained from the fleshy leaves of several species of aloe, a plant native to Africa but now cultivated in various parts of the world for its medicinal properties. Its purgative action was known to the ancient Greeks, but especially in the nineteenth century it began to be widely used in most European countries. It is even slower in action than the other members of this group, taking usually over 12 hours to induce purgation. It is more liable to produce pelvic congestion than the other anthracene purgatives; it also tends to stimulate the uterus after absorption. It is therefore usually avoided in pregnant women, though the danger of causing abortion is slight with ordinary doses. It is a favourite ingredient of proprietary medicines. It is conveniently prescribed in pill or tablet form. The dose of **Powdered Aloes**, B.P., is 0·12–0·3 G. (2–5 gr.). An active principle, **Aloin**, B.P., 15–60 mg. ($\frac{1}{4}$–1 gr.), does not seem superior to crude aloes.

Rhubarb, B.P., is the dried rhizome of *Rheum palmatum*, a plant somewhat resembling garden rhubarb, which grows in China and Tibet. Its medicinal properties were known to the Chinese earlier than 2000 B.C., and it has been imported for centuries into western countries. Unlike the other members of this group, rhubarb contains (in addition to its purgative principle) tannic acid (p. 52) which has an astringent action. It tends therefore to produce some constipation after purgation and hence is not suitable for repeated administration, e.g. in chronic constipation. It is chiefly used in dyspepsia or diarrhoea due to the presence of undigested material in the alimentary canal. It is often prescribed for children. Of the official preparations, one of the most commonly used is **Compound Powder of Rhubarb**, B.P., 0·6–4 G. (10–60 gr.). This powder is often called Gregory's Powder from Dr. James Gregory (1753–1821), an Edinburgh physician, who first prescribed it. It contains, besides Rhubarb, Heavy and Light Magnesium Carbonate which seem to increase the action of rhubarb, and Ginger, which tends to prevent griping. A drawback to the powder is its disagreeable taste and smell, which it is difficult to conceal. The B.P. contains also a **Compound Tincture of Rhubarb**. The U.S.P. has discarded rhubarb.

Phenolphthalein, B.P., U.S.P., a synthetic substance, may be taken with the anthracene group, which it resembles in type of action. It acts chiefly on the large intestine and takes from 6 to 12 hours to act. It is insoluble in water, but is dissolved by bile and alkali in the intestine and produces purgation by mild irritation. Some of it may be absorbed and re-excreted in the intestine, and so its purgative action may last for a few days. It is partly excreted in the urine, to which, if alkaline, it may give a pink colour. In some people phenolphthalein has provoked a peculiar eruption of the skin which may last for months. It is usually given as **Tablets of Phenolphthalein**, B.P., 60–300 mg. (1–5 gr.), U.S.P., 60 mg.

Other purgatives dealt with elsewhere are salines (p. 44) and mercurials (p. 63).

In the case of all the purgatives mentioned above, the remedies are given by mouth. Accumulations of faeces in the large intestine can, however, also be got rid of by injections of fluids (*enemas*) into the rectum. An enema of a pint of warm water alone may be used, and acts partly by distending the lower bowel and so provoking peristaltic contraction, and partly by softening the scybala. The action may be increased by adding a slight irritant such as turpentine or soap to the water. Oil or glycerin may be used for a similar purpose. *Glycerin*, B.P., acts by withdrawing water from the mucous membrane of the rectum and inducing peristalsis by the resulting irritation. For this purpose it can conveniently be dispensed in the form of a suppository. *Suppositories of Glycerin*, B.P., are made by incorporating Glycerin with Gelatine which imparts enough rigidity for insertion but liquefies at the rectal temperature.

Drugs can also be given by parenteral injection to stimulate intestinal movements, e.g. physostigmine (p. 158), certain choline esters (p. 157), or pituitary extract (p. 180).

For the relief of colic or to prevent griping, volatile oils (p. 43), hyoscyamus (p. 160), or, in special cases, pethidine (meperidine) (p. 120) may be used.

VEGETABLE ASTRINGENTS: TANNINS

Tannins occur in a great variety of plants, ranging from herbs to trees, belonging to different natural orders and found in all parts of the world. Extracts of some of these plants have come to be of great commercial importance from their use in industries, especially of tanning and dyeing. In the process of tanning, the proteins of hides are precipitated by the tannic acid in the plant extract. The tissue (leather) thus becomes hard, dry, and resistant to putrefaction, while retaining much of its flexibility. Some of the plants containing tannic acid have come into medicinal use, and in this case they act also by precipitating proteins. There are slight differences between the tannins of different plants which influence to some extent their therapeutic uses.

Tannic Acid, B.P., (Tannin), is obtained from oak-galls, as a light brownish powder, freely soluble in water, with a characteristic odour, a strongly astringent taste, and an acid reaction.

Solutions of tannic acid precipitate proteins and thus, when applied to a mucous membrane or raw surface, coagulate a film on the surface of the cells. This film acts as a protective to an inflamed surface and also lessens the passage of fluids through the superficial membrane. Tannic acid can thus be used for a variety of conditions as an astringent, acting physically in the same way as solutions of metallic salts.

In the mouth tannic acid produces, in addition to a harsh bitter taste, a feeling of dryness and roughness due to coagulation of the superficial layers of protein. It is used for tonsillitis and relaxed sore throat. It also checks bleeding from the gums. This it does by coagulating the blood proteins and so favouring the formation of normal clotting. For exerting its action on the mouth and throat the *Glycerin of Tannic Acid*, B.P., may be employed as a paint or diluted as a gargle.

When swallowed, tannic acid exerts an astringent action on the stomach and intestine and tends to produce constipation. Many tannin-containing plants, such as catechu were formerly used in the treatment of diarrhoea but they were not very effective and are no longer official. *Hamamelis*, B.P. (Witch Hazel Leaves), is used to furnish preparations which are applied externally as weak astringents.

V

HEAVY METALS

JUST as the heavy metals have certain chemical resemblances whereby they form a group, so one might expect that they would have some common pharmacological properties. These similarities they display especially in their local actions but also to some extent in a common pattern of toxic effects if they are absorbed in sufficient quantity. It is convenient to consider these actions so far as they are common to metallic salts and thereafter to take up the metals individually.

LOCAL ACTIONS OF HEAVY METALS

When a soluble salt of heavy metal is added to a solution of albumin, a precipitate is formed which is the albuminate of the metal. Protein, which is amphoteric, acts in this reaction as an acid, forming an insoluble salt of the metal. There are three pharmacological actions obtainable from such metallic salts which depend upon this interaction with proteins, viz. astringent, caustic, and antiseptic actions. Of these, the astringent action depends solely upon the actual physical coagulation of the proteins, whereas the caustic and antiseptic actions are due at least as much to the toxic action of the metals on the cells, independent of whether the protein is coagulated or not.

ASTRINGENT. When a solution of heavy metal is applied to a mucous membrane, a film of the surface is coagulated. If the solution be strong, this may lead to an opacity of the surface which may be obvious on inspection. When a stick of solid silver nitrate is drawn across the red granulating surface of a wound, it leaves a white wake of coagulation, giving the appearance as if one had drawn a white chalk over a red surface. When a dilute solution of silver nitrate is applied to a mucous membrane, the coagulation of proteins will not be so intense and no change in the surface may be apparent to naked-eye observation. At least two effects may result from this coagulation of the surface film of the cells. In the first place the surface may be drawn together, puckered in fact, and this was the original meaning of the word astringent. In the second place the permeability of the cell surface will be altered. If a solution of lead acetate or of tannic acid, either of which coagulates proteins, be applied to a mucus-secreting surface, it may be seen that the cells become more opaque and the secretion of the mucus diminishes. One of the chief uses of astringents is to produce this effect of diminishing exudation or secretion from mucous membranes or raw surfaces.

CAUSTIC. So long as this coagulation of the surface film of the cells is not too intense, it can be imagined that the effects will be confined to those changes in permeability already described. The interchange of substances necessary for the life of the cell can still take place through the unaltered deep surfaces of the cells. If, however, the coagulation is too intense, or if the metal penetrates to the cell nucleus, the cell may die. In this case the metallic salt exerts a 'caustic' action, that is to say there is an actual destruction of cells and the dead cells are shed off. The difference between astringent and caustic action may be therefore one only of degree.

ANTISEPTIC. So far, the results of the application of a metallic salt have been considered only from the point of view of the tissue-cells. If, however, there be a bacterial infection of the surface, the proteins of the bacterial cell will be subject to the same changes as the proteins of the tissue-cells; and as the entire surface of a bacterium may be exposed to the solution, it may presumably be more seriously endangered than the tissue-cells which are exposed on one side only.

Actually, however, even in superficial bacterial infections, the micro-organisms are more or less embedded in the tissues, so that bacteria and tissue-cells are almost equally exposed to the antiseptic solution. It is therefore difficult, with metallic solutions and indeed with most antiseptics, to find a concentration that will inhibit bacterial growth without doing some damage to the tissue-cells.

As these local actions depend upon interaction between metallic ion and protein, the intensity of this action will vary with the degree of ionization and the solubility of the salt employed. Insoluble metallic compounds may also combine with proteins, but more slowly and less completely. Such insoluble compounds therefore exert much feebler, but sometimes more prolonged, local actions.

OLIGODYNAMIC ACTION OF METALS. Very low concentrations of most metallic salts (1 in 1 million or more) may exert an antiseptic action, especially in the absence of organic matter. The multiplication of bacteria is stopped and, if sufficient time be allowed, they may be killed. The metal is adsorbed into the bacterium, giving a rising concentration in it. The action of insoluble metallic salts and oxides is probably due to this type of action arising from slow liberation of ionized metal.

METALLIC POISONING

Some metals are, under ordinary conditions of medicinal use, not absorbed at all or at least not to a degree sufficient to produce recognizable effects, but most metals and the metalloids (see Chap. VI) if absorbed in sufficient quantity exert toxic effects which conform more or less to a common pattern. These may be acute or chronic and the organs most affected are the liver (hepatitis), the skin (dermatitis), and the central nervous system (encephalopathy). In addition the metals are concentrated at the points of excretion and may thus cause colic (spasm of the large intestine) or nephrosis (damage to the kidney tubules). The reason for the common pattern of toxicity, which varies in severity and site with the different metals and with the amount, is the property which metals exhibit of combining with labile —SH groups which are present in various cellular enzymes. This binding or 'chelating' power is reversible and metal poisoning can thus be treated by administration of an excess of available sulphydril, usually in the form of *Dimercaprol*, B.P., $CH_2(SH) \cdot CH(SH) \cdot CH_2OH$. This compound is most effective in reversing tissue damage from metals and bringing about their excretion in the urine. It is a valuable antidote in poisoning due to copper, zinc, silver, gold, bismuth, and arsenic, but of less value in lead poisoning because its effect is short-lived and the soluble lead complex formed is itself toxic.

Dimercaprol was first used in ointment form as an antidote to the blistering arsenical war gas Lewisite, hence its original name of British Anti-Lewisite and the now familiar synonym initials B.A.L. It is usually given as *Injection of Dimercaprol*, B.P., a sterile 5 per cent. solution in Benzyl Benzoate and Arachis Oil, administered intramuscularly, 4 ml. in divided doses during the first day and subsequently in accordance with the needs of the patient.

COPPER

Copper Sulphate, B.P., is the most important salt of copper. It is freely soluble in water and the solution is acid. It has the local actions already described as characteristic of soluble salts of heavy metals. It is caustic in solid form, or in very concentrated solution. Weaker solutions are astringent and antiseptic. It is used chiefly as an antiseptic and astringent for mucous membranes, such as the conjunctiva. Internally copper sulphate is sometimes used as an emetic. It irritates the stomach by combining with the proteins of the mucous membrane, and provokes vomiting reflexly through the vomiting centre. In prescribing it as an emetic certain conditions have to be complied with which have to be observed also in the use of any emetic which acts by irritation. It should be prescribed in solution (if dry, it will have a caustic action on the oesophagus and stomach); if too strong, the solution will produce undue irritation; if too weak, it will not produce sufficient to cause vomiting. A suitable strength is about 1 per cent. and the emetic dose, 0·3–0·6 G. (5–10 gr.), should be given in such dilution.

Copper sulphate has a special use in phosphorus poisoning. It forms an insoluble and almost inert phosphide of copper which checks the local actions, and delays the absorption of phosphorus.

Copper facilitates the full use of iron in the formation of haemoglobin. Only traces of it are needed in adults and even the poorest diets provide enough for the purpose. Exceptionally in certain cases of nutritional hypochromic anaemia in infancy, copper is alleged to enhance the remedial effect of iron.

ZINC

Zinc Sulphate, B.P., U.S.P., has actions almost identical with those of copper sulphate but is less irritant. It is used as an antiseptic for the eye in solutions of 0·1 to 1·0 per cent. according to the condition. Internally it can be used as a reflex emetic in doses of 0·6–2 G. (10–30 gr.).

In addition to this soluble salt, certain insoluble salts, especially the Oxide and Stearate, are also used. Being insoluble, they combine only slowly with proteins, and consequently exert a less energetic but more prolonged local action than the soluble salts. They are chiefly used as astringents and antiseptics, in lotions and ointments, for skin diseases. For this purpose there are several official preparations including an Ointment and a Cream. The *Paste of Zinc Oxide and Salicylic Acid*, B.P. (Lassar's Paste), is much used.

Calamine, B.P., a zinc carbonate coloured pink by addition of iron oxide, acts like zinc oxide and can impart a pinkish colour to ointments and lotions, as in the official Lotion.

ALUMINIUM

The salts of aluminium have actions similar to those of copper and zinc. *Alum*, B.P., is a double sulphate of aluminium with either potassium or ammonium. It is used locally as an astringent antiseptic.

Light Kaolin, B.P., is a native aluminium silicate. It can be obtained as a fine, soft powder, insoluble in water. It is given in diarrhoeas and cholera. Here the effect is due not to any specific effect of aluminium but to the fact that the powder, being inert owing to its insolubility, can be given in large doses, 15–60 G. ($\frac{1}{2}$–2 oz.), and the fine particles adsorb toxins in the intestine and also act as a protective to the mucous membrane. Kaolin thus acts much in the same way as insoluble bismuth salts (p. 68).

It has a similar protective action on irritated or abraded skin surfaces, when used as a dusting powder.

Heavy Kaolin, B.P., is used to make *Kaolin Poultice*, B.P. This preparation contains also Glycerin (which retains water) as well as antiseptic substances, e.g. Boric Acid and Methyl Salicylate. It is applied hot and has the merit of keeping warm and damp for a long time.

SILVER

Silver Nitrate, B.P., is the only official soluble salt of silver. It forms a dense coagulum with proteins and is also precipitated by the chlorides in the tissues. Its astringent action is therefore powerful but superficial. Concentrated solutions are caustic, but, for the same reasons, not penetrating. Silver nitrate is also a powerful antiseptic.

Externally it is used in dilute solution as an astringent-antiseptic. It is of value as an application to mucous membranes, such as the conjunctiva. The strength of solution used varies with the sensitiveness of the surface to which it is applied, and ranges from 0·02 to 2·0 per cent. The *Silver Nitrate Ophthalmic Solution*, U.S.P., contains 1 per cent. It is used commonly in the form of a solid stick, *Toughened Silver Nitrate*, B.P., as a caustic, possessing the advantage that its extent of action can be limited.

It has no astringent action on the intestine, as it is precipitated in the stomach as silver chloride and reduced to metallic silver in the intestine.

COLLOIDAL COMPOUNDS OF SILVER

One disadvantage attending the use of silver nitrate as an astringent or antiseptic is the amount of irritation it produces, due to its combining with the proteins of the tissues. To obviate this, compounds have been introduced in which the silver is already united with protein, so that little of the silver is in an ionizable form to unite with the tissue protein. Such compounds are much less irritating than silver nitrate, but, as the antiseptic action is also dependent upon ionizable silver, they are also less antiseptic. For some purposes, e.g. for infections of the eye and urethra, they are preferable to silver nitrate itself.

The B.P. has *Silver Protein* containing 8 per cent. of silver.

LEAD

Lead Acetate, B.P., is the only official soluble salt of lead. It differs from the soluble salts of the metals previously considered chiefly in being less irritant and having less antiseptic power. It is, however, an active astringent, producing a dense precipitation of proteins. As it is also precipitated by chlorides in the tissues, its action is superficial, which is usually desirable in an astringent. Solutions of acetate of lead are applied for their astringent and sedative action to the skin.

Chronic lead poisoning

Lead can, if it gains entrance into the body in small amounts over long periods, produce chronic poisoning. Of the commoner causes may be mentioned the drinking of water, beer, or cider contaminated with lead, or the swallowing or inhalation of lead in some form by lead workers, plumbers, compositors, or painters. In nearly all cases small quantities of lead compounds have been ingested or inhaled (as powder) for a considerable time, and, though absorption is slow and incomplete, excretion is even less rapid, and the metal accumulates in the tissues, giving rise to toxic effects.

Among the early and fairly constant symptoms are loss of appetite, constipation, and the appearance of a blue line at the margin of the gums due to the formation there of sulphide of lead. A peculiar basophilic change in the red blood corpuscles often occurs early, and is very significant of lead poisoning.

The nervous system, both central and peripheral, is especially prone to be attacked by lead. The most common result of this is peripheral neuritis, which usually first affects the nerves supplying the extensors of the wrists and fingers but spares the brachio-radialis, 'wrist drop'. Sometimes the muscles of the foot and other muscles are affected. The sensory nerves may be also affected, giving rise to areas of hyperaesthesia or anaesthesia.

Lead has also a stimulant action on smooth muscle, giving rise to three effects of importance—colic due to spasmodic contraction of the intestinal muscle, uterine contractions which may lead to abortion, and arteriosclerotic changes sometimes with high blood pressure.

The treatment of chronic lead poisoning consists in stopping further absorption of lead and accelerating the excretion of lead stored in the tissues. Lead is largely deposited in the bones, and its excretion may be hastened (but not too quickly, as the increase of lead in the blood may temporarily aggravate the symptoms) by administration of parathyroid extract, potassium iodide, or ammonium chloride.

MERCURY

Mercury has been used medicinally in the form not only of mercuric and mercurous compounds but also of preparations of metallic mercury itself. However combined, mercury always exerts qualitatively the same action, but the intensity and rapidity of action are modified by the degree of solubility and dissociation of the particular compound used. Thus the local actions of mercury are much more rapidly and energetically displayed by the perchloride, which is soluble, than by the subchloride, which is insoluble.

Local actions

It is convenient first to consider the action of a soluble mercuric salt like the perchloride. *Mercuric Chloride*, B.P., or corrosive sublimate ($HgCl_2$) is soluble 1 in 16 in water. It precipitates proteins, but this precipitate is more readily soluble in excess of protein than are the albuminates of most heavy metals. Hence solutions of corrosive sublimate are almost non-astringent, because no permanent coagulum is formed. Moreover, whereas depth of local action of soluble silver and lead salts is prevented by their precipitation as chlorides, this does not happen with corrosive sublimate, which is itself a soluble chloride. The latter is therefore a much more penetrating caustic, so that the depth of action is difficult to control. Hence mercury is rarely used medicinally as an astringent or caustic. *Mercuric Chloride* is a powerful antiseptic, generally used in the concentrations of 1 in 20,000 to 1 in 2,000, but it has been largely supplanted by better antiseptics and is no longer official in the U.S.P.

Other soluble salts of mercury act similarly, their activity depending greatly upon the degree of ionization, mercuric cyanide, which dissociates slightly, being a feebler antiseptic than mercuric chloride, which dissociates readily. Insoluble salts of mercury combine much more slowly with proteins and exercise a weaker but more prolonged antiseptic action.

Organic compounds of mercury, in which the mercury does not ionize, are also used as antiseptics. One such compound, *Phenylmercuric Nitrate*, B.P., has a special use for preserving solutions or suspensions for parenteral injection. It is added to these in a concentration of 0·002 per cent. before the solution is sterilized by heating.

These compounds show corresponding differences in the intensity of their local actions on the alimentary canal. Thus the soluble perchloride is a severe irritant, producing diarrhoea in small doses, whereas much larger doses of calomel are required to produce this effect. The dose of Mercuric Chloride given in the B.P. 1948 was 2–4 mg. ($\frac{1}{32}$–$\frac{1}{16}$ gr.), whereas that of Mercurous Chloride (calomel), B.P., is 30–200 mg. ($\frac{1}{2}$–3 gr.). That fifty times as much of the latter can be given as of the former is due to its insolubility, and is in spite of the fact that it contains, weight for weight, more mercury than the perchloride.

Mercury is, compared with the metals previously considered, readily absorbed. It tends to be stored in the body, especially in the kidneys and liver, and part of the absorbed mercury is excreted very slowly. It is eliminated by nearly all excreting glands, especially by the kidneys and by the gut, but also in the saliva, milk, &c. Owing to the slowness of its excretion it is liable to accumulate in the body and to produce toxic effects if given continuously. Usually, in small doses, it excites to greater activity the glands by which it is excreted. Single medicinal doses usually produce no marked effects, except possibly diarrhoea and increased diuresis. Beyond these effects it is chiefly the toxicology of mercury that is important, namely the toxic effects produced by a single large dose or by long-continued small doses.

Mercury poisoning

In *acute poisoning* by ingestion of a soluble salt like the perchloride, the symptoms come on within a few minutes—pain in the throat, gullet, and abdomen with frequent vomiting and purging, the evacuations being usually streaked with blood. Symptoms of collapse follow, of the usual type consequent upon corrosive irritation of the alimentary canal. Death may occur in a few hours, but usually in from one to five days, and occasionally even later. When death is delayed the symptoms merge into those of chronic poisoning due to absorption of mercury, suppression of urine due to nephritis being the main cause of a fatal issue.

Chronic poisoning from continued absorption of small quantities may occur. An early symptom is increased salivation, probably due to irritation of the salivary glands by the mercury which they excrete. The amount of saliva secreted may be enormous. Soreness of the gums, loosening of the teeth, and even gangrene of the cheek may also occur. There are often present also symptoms of irritation of the stomach and intestine, loss of appetite, nausea, and diarrhoea.

The urine may be at first increased, but later nephritis is often set up with albuminuria. Especially in the late stages of acute poisoning there may be marked diminution, or even complete suppression, of the urine. Actual necrosis of the kidney epithelium may be induced, with deposit of calcium phosphate and carbonate in the necrosed cells.

Skin rashes not uncommonly occur with mercury, most frequently when it is applied externally, but also from any other method of administration. In workers with mercury, a kind of chronic poisoning may arise which is usually ushered in by symptoms of subacute poisoning, but which eventually affects chiefly the central nervous system. The chief symptoms are tremor of certain muscles, usually affecting the muscles of the face and hands first, and consisting of fine movements aggravated by voluntary effort. Later, the movements may become continuous and epileptiform in nature. Various sensory disturbances have also been described, as well as a peculiar type of nervous irritability (erethismus mercurialis).

Pink disease, a prolonged and serious condition occurring usually in late infancy, has been found to be related to ingestion of mercury, which, especially as calomel, has long been used empirically in 'teething powders'. Since the use of such powders has been strongly denounced, pink disease has become a rarity.

Therapeutic uses of Mercury

Compounds of mercury have a wide use as *antiseptics*. Soluble salts, like perchloride, are used to disinfect the hands, &c., but they are irritant to delicate tissues, such as serous membranes, and they corrode steel instruments. Insoluble preparations are used in the form of lotions and ointments as antiseptics for syphilitic lesions, skin diseases, &c. **Ointment of Ammoniated Mercury**, B.P., is used in skin infections, and the milder **Eye Ointment of Mercuric Oxide**, B.P., in eye conditions. There are many other official preparations of mercury for external use as antiseptics.

Internally mercury in the form of **Mercurous Chloride**, B.P., (Calomel), 30–200 mg. ($\frac{1}{2}$–3 gr.), is used as a *purgative* and intestinal antiseptic.

Calomel has long been used as a *diuretic*, especially in cases of dropsy due to heart disease. In recent years some organic compounds of mercury have been found to be far more effective for this purpose (p. 26).

Mercury has been used in the treatment of syphilis for over four centuries, but has been superseded in recent years by more effective and less toxic remedies, e.g. neoarsphenamine, bismuth, and penicillin.

IRON

Iron differs from the other heavy metals in being an important normal constituent of the body. In mammals most of the iron is contained in the haemoglobin of the blood and is essential for its formation, but traces of iron are found in all tissues and are probably necessary for the life of all cells.

LOCAL ACTIONS OF IRON SALTS. Ferric chloride precipitates proteins, but solutions of it are too acid and irritating for general use as astringents or antiseptics. They are occasionally used for the local arrest of haemorrhage, which they tend to bring about by coagulating the proteins of the blood and thus favouring the development of normal clotting. When given by mouth it has of course no effect on distal bleeding, e.g. from the lung or kidney. Ferrous salts and the 'scale' preparations are less astringent than ferric.

GENERAL ACTIONS OF IRON. When iron salts are given by mouth, most of the iron passes unabsorbed through the alimentary canal; and the small amounts that are absorbed are insufficient to produce any immediate effect or indeed any measurable effect unless in cases of iron deficiency. For practical purposes, therefore, the pharmacology of iron resolves itself into the action of iron in abnormal conditions of iron metabolism, especially in deficiency of haemoglobin.

The total amount of iron in the body of an adult man is about 4·5 G., about two-thirds of it being in haemoglobin. There is a continual and inevitable, though small, daily excretion of iron, resulting indirectly, for example, from the continual destruction of red blood corpuscles. This amount is about 1 mg., most of which is excreted in the bile and by the large intestine (through the mucous membrane), but traces are found also in the urine. Though this daily loss of iron is small, it must be remembered that it is considerable in proportion to the total iron of the body. This excretion is, however, compensated by the absorption of iron from the food. As iron is a necessary constituent of most vegetable and animal tissues, it follows that nearly all foods contain it in small quantities. As iron is essential for the life of mammals, it goes without saying that the amount of iron in the food is normally adequate, otherwise the animals could not have survived in this dependence. The amount in the daily diet will obviously depend upon the amount and nature of the food, but the interesting point is that a normal well-regulated diet does not contain any enormous excess of iron. It has been estimated at about 10 mg. per day. An ill-balanced diet, especially if deficient in meat or vegetables, may easily contain too little iron, and in such cases it is important to make good this deficiency by administering iron salts. Iron is absorbed by the small intestine only as the ferrous ion, absorption being aided by the acidity of the contents. It is then altered to ferric iron during combination with a protein iron-acceptor in the mucosal cell called apoferritin, to form ferritin. This mechanism is easily saturated, whereupon absorption ceases and only becomes active again as the serum iron level falls. Iron is normally stored in all tissues but perhaps largely in liver, spleen, and muscle, as ferritin, from which store the serum iron is replenished and iron transported to the bone marrow; there it is synthesized to haemoglobin and included in the red blood cells. Transport of iron from ferritin stores in mucosa or tissue is by combination with serum globulin. Effete red blood cells are destroyed in the spleen, liver, &c., and most of the iron conserved as tissue ferritin, the pigmented moiety of haemoglobin being excreted as bile pigment. At this point a little iron is lost also. It follows that a patient may exhibit normal blood haemoglobin levels (15·5 G. per 100 ml.) but have low tissue iron stores, and that absorption of administered iron may be poor because serum iron remains high and mucosal apoferritin is saturated. It also follows that absorption of an iron-containing medicament decreases as the mucosal apoferritin gets taken up and as the blood and tissue levels rise and that medication in iron-deficiency anaemia needs to be prolonged. The amount excreted is slight and is not capable of increase so that toxic effects result if too much iron should gain entry to the body.

Therapeutic uses of Iron Salts

The chief use of iron salts is in iron-deficient anaemias in which the red cells are hypochromic (undercoloured) or microcytic (undersized). There is a reduction in the number of red cells with a disproportionate reduction in the percentage of haemoglobin. That is to say, each red cell contains less than the normal proportion of haemoglobin. One form of this anaemia, chlorosis—so called from the greenish (Greek *chloros*) colour of the skin seen in advanced cases—was formerly common in adolescent females but has become less frequent and less severe in the last half-century. More important now are the hypochromic anaemias of pregnancy. An increased loss of iron occurs during menstruation and many women enter on pregnancy with low iron reserves. During pregnancy iron must be provided for the needs of the foetus as well as of the mother. Mere determination of the haemoglobin level does not always reveal iron deficiency, for the iron reserves may be severely depleted before haemoglobin values are affected. This masked reduction of iron in the tissues and in the iron-containing enzymes may adversely affect both mother and child. It is important that women should be watched during pregnancy to ensure that they are receiving and utilizing sufficient iron. An existing anaemia may be aggravated by loss of blood during labour, and, if a mother nurses her baby, lactation takes an additional toll of her iron reserves. Anaemia must be guarded against during this period also.

Infants may require supplementary iron, as milk is poor in

iron. Medicinal iron may also be needed by rapidly growing children or in convalescence from various diseases. In such conditions the improvement in the blood takes time. The formed red cells cannot synthesize haemoglobin. The rise in the percentage of haemoglobin can occur only from the formation of new red cells, containing an increased amount of haemo-globin, gradually replacing the hypochromic red cells which are normally and regularly being destroyed, the average life of a red cell being calculated as 120 days. To complete this re-placement process usually takes weeks.

The great majority of cases of hypochromic anaemia can be successfully treated by administration of iron salts by mouth. These tend to irritate the stomach and should therefore be taken after meals. Those now most commonly used are *Ferrous Sulphate*, B.P., U.S.P., 0·2–0·3 G. (3–5 gr.), or the *Tablets of Exsiccated Ferrous Sulphate*, B.P., 60–200 mg. (1–3 gr.), or a 'scale' preparation *Ferric Ammonium Citrate*, B.P., 1–3 G. (15–45 gr.). More recently *Ferrous Gluconate*, B.P., U.S.P., which is less irritant has been much used, 0·3–0·6 G. (5–10 gr.). When iron is not well tolerated by mouth or when it is not sufficiently absorbed, it may be given parenterally. A preparation of iron and dextran given by intramuscular in-jection produces little irritation and may rapidly restore the haemoglobin. Exceptionally a saccharated iron oxide has been used by intravenous injection but is more likely to produce toxic effects.

VI

METALLOIDS

IT is convenient to take together a group which includes bismuth, antimony, and arsenic. They form a series which closely resemble the heavy metals and are often included among the heavy metals proper.

BISMUTH

Most official salts of bismuth are insoluble in water, and they do not therefore have the immediate precipitant action on proteins and the resulting local actions which are characteristic of the soluble salts of the heavy metals. The local actions of salts of bismuth are indeed largely dependent on the fact that these salts occur in the form of very fine insoluble powders. These are used externally as dusting powders and internally as sedatives in dyspepsias and diarrhoeas. They act mechanically by coating over the surfaces and possibly also by adsorbing toxins. When given by mouth, only traces of bismuth are absorbed—not enough to produce general effects; the faeces may be coloured grey or black from formation of bismuth sulphide, which is black.

The salts most commonly used for oral administration are *Bismuth Carbonate*, B.P., 0·6–2 G. (10–30 gr.), *Bismuth Subcarbonate*, U.S.P., 1–4 Gm., and *Bismuth Salicylate*, B.P., 0·6–2 G. (10–30 gr.).

Bismuth compounds have been extensively used in the treatment of syphilis. They have now supplanted mercury as they are less toxic and have a more rapid curative action. Arsenical compounds (p. 73) must usually be supplemented by bismuth, but all these metals have been largely superseded by antibiotics in the treatment of syphilis. Not being absorbed from the alimentary canal, bismuth must be given by intramuscular injection, as a suspension of an insoluble salt like the oxychloride, e.g. *Injection of Bismuth Oxychloride*, B.P., which is a sterile suspension containing 0·2 G. in 2 ml., given in doses of 1 to 2 ml. (15 to 30 min.). A similar *Bismuth Subsalicylate Injection* is official in the U.S.P.

Such injections form pockets of the insoluble metal or its salt in the muscle, from which bismuth is slowly absorbed. The concentration of bismuth in the blood is very low, but sufficient to affect the spirochaetes.

Soluble double salts of bismuth, e.g. *Bismuth Sodium Tartrate*, B.P., are also used. Though this salt is soluble, it is precipitated in the muscular tissues and the effect is much the same as with an insoluble salt, though a solution may spread more than a suspension and so provide a larger area for absorption of the precipitated particles. Watery or oily suspensions may be used, the latter causing less local pain. Owing to the slow and prolonged absorption, injections need be given only once a week.

The chief symptoms of chronic poisoning are nausea, albuminuria, ulceration of the gums, a dark patchy discoloration of the mouth, and jaundice.

ANTIMONY

Antimony, in the form of tartar emetic, has had a chequered career as a therapeutic agent. From the early part of the seventeenth century onwards it was used for a great variety of diseases, in many of which its value was hotly disputed. During the nineteenth century its reputation waned, but in this century new and established therapeutic uses for it have been discovered.

Antimony Potassium Tartrate, B.P., U.S.P., or tartar emetic, forms colourless crystals or a white powder with a disagreeable metallic taste, soluble 1 in 17 of cold water.

Tartar emetic is an irritant even to the skin, but more so to mucous membranes. Taken internally in doses of 30–60 mg. ($\frac{1}{2}$–1 gr.), it produces reflex emesis, from irritation of the gastric mucous membrane. Vomiting does not usually occur before 20–30 minutes, and is apt to be repeated. The usual concomitants of nausea, especially increased bronchial and sweat secretion, are conspicuously exhibited. These secondary effects of gastric irritation can be produced by doses too small to produce actual vomiting, and in such doses, 2–8 mg. ($\frac{1}{32}$–$\frac{1}{8}$ gr.), tartar emetic is sometimes used as an expectorant and diaphoretic.

So far as these actions are concerned it might therefore have become by now a superfluous remedy, had it not in recent years been discovered to possess a singular and specific remedial effect in certain infections. The beginning of this new phase in its history was the discovery that antimony has a powerful trypanocidal action. Owing to its local irritant action, tartar emetic cannot be given by mouth or subcutaneously in sufficient quantity to be effective. It was found, however, that it can be given successfully by intravenous injection. Other remedies have been found more effective in trypanosomiasis but, when it was established that tartar emetic could safely be given intravenously, this method of administration was tried in other types of infection and it was found that antimony has a wide range of anti-parasitic activity.

One group of diseases, all caused by infections with different species of protozoal parasites of the genus *Leishmania*, e.g. kala-azar and oriental sore, have proved amenable to treatment with antimony. Another group of diseases, due to an entirely different type of infective organism, schistosomiasis (bilharziasis), may yield also to antimony therapy (p. 309). These diseases cannot be cured by a single injection and require a course of graded and spaced doses until a suitable total amount has been given. With antimony potassium tartrate or the corresponding sodium salt, *Antimony Sodium Tartrate*, B.P., such a course may begin with a dose of 30 mg. ($\frac{1}{2}$ gr.), increasing to 120 mg. (2 gr.) and given thrice a week intravenously.

Many new synthetic compounds have been prepared and tested. Of well-established compounds may be mentioned *Stibophen*, B.P., U.S.P., 0·1–0·3 G., a catechol disulphonate compound of antimony used especially in schistosomiasis, and *Sodium Antimonylgluconate*. These compounds can be given intramuscularly as well as intravenously and are less toxic than tartar emetic. In these two compounds antimony is *trivalent*.

For the diseases mentioned some *pentavalent* compounds of antimony, e.g. **Sodium Stibogluconate**, have proved especially useful in the treatment of kala-azar.

Intravenous injections of antimony compounds may produce, among other symptoms, cough, pains in the shoulder and abdomen, and more rarely pneumonia.

ARSENIC

The modern use of arsenic as a therapeutic agent began substantially with the publication in 1786 by Thomas Fowler (1736–1801), a physician of Stafford, of *Medical Reports on the Effects of Arsenic in the Cure of Agues*, &c., and with the aid of an apothecary, Hughes, he compounded a substitute, Liquor Arsenicalis (still called Fowler's Solution), for the quack remedy then known as 'Tasteless Ague or Fever Drops'. A century and a half has elapsed since Fowler's work was published, and in that time preparations of arsenic have been tried in a great variety of diseases. During this century, until largely superseded by antibiotics such as penicillin, organic compounds of arsenic were of great importance in the treatment of syphilis and trypanosomiasis.

Arsenic Trioxide, B.P., As_2O_3, occurs usually in the form of a white power or porcelain-like masses. It dissolves slowly in rather less than 100 parts of cold water. It is almost tasteless and odourless.

Arsenic trioxide is a caustic. It does not combine with proteins like the heavy metals, and its caustic action is slower than that of corrosive sublimate, for example.

Arsenic Poisoning

ACUTE POISONING. As one would expect of a caustic substance, arsenic trioxide causes severe irritation of the stomach and intestine, with vomiting and profuse and repeated watery diarrhoea. Secondary symptoms supervene, resulting from the rapid loss of fluid and the dilatation of the abdominal vessels, e.g. thirst, diminution or suppression of urine, low blood pressure, and collapse, with coldness and pallor of the skin, and rapid, feeble pulse. In acute fatal poisoning, death may occur within twenty-four hours, but is usually postponed for two or three days, when the patient dies of exhaustion. If the dose is smaller than the lethal dose, recovery may occur without symptoms other than those described, but more or less marked symptoms due to absorbed arsenic are also apt to occur. If the quantity absorbed be large, fatty degeneration of the liver and other organs is a usual result.

CHRONIC POISONING. When smaller quantities are ingested over long periods, chronic poisoning due to absorbed arsenic may ensue. The following are among the common effects of chronic poisoning. There may be dyspepsia, nausea, or diarrhoea. An important early diagnostic symptom is redness and itching of the conjunctiva, and a catarrhal condition of the upper air passages, with sneezing or coughing. A variety of skin eruptions may occur, and the epidermis may be shed off in fine brownish scales or flakes. A leaden-coloured pigmentation of the skin is not uncommon. Usually at a later period, symptoms may appear from peripheral neuritis. This may affect sensory nerves, causing various disturbances of sensation, and also motor nerves, producing paralysis of voluntary muscles, the first sign of which is usually disappearance of the ankle-jerk. If the ingestion of arsenic is stopped, recovery may be complete, but not, of course, if the muscles have degenerated.

Arsenic is excreted slowly, some of it within a day or two in the faeces, but much of it is stored for an indefinite time in the tissues, and eliminated in the hair, epidermis, &c.

THERAPEUTIC USES OF ARSENIC. *Arsenic Trioxide*, B.P., has been used empirically in the treatment of many, generally chronic, diseases, usually with doubtful benefit. It is still sometimes used in chronic superficial skin diseases, e.g. psoriasis. The preparation chiefly used is *Arsenical Solution*, B.P. (Fowler's Solution), 0·12–0·5 ml. (2–8 min.), which contains 1 per cent. of Arsenic Trioxide.

ORGANIC COMPOUNDS OF ARSENIC

Though in recent years there has been a decline in the medicinal use of inorganic preparations of arsenic, this has been more than compensated by the extensive employment of organic compounds of arsenic, especially in diseases due to trypanosomes and allied organisms. Arsenic was known to have some effect in syphilis and malaria, and when sleeping sickness and many other diseases were shown to be due to protozoal parasites, inorganic arsenic was tried in them. It proved, however, too poisonous to the patient to be of much value. Later an extensive series of investigations was begun on the action of organic compounds of arsenic in these diseases, with a view to discovery of some compound that would be less toxic to the host but more toxic to the parasite than inorganic arsenic.

The first important compound to be used was atoxyl, or the sodium salt of arsanilic acid. This was tried with some success in sleeping sickness, but was found to produce serious toxic actions, e.g. blindness. Ehrlich showed that atoxyl had no toxic action on trypanosomes *in vitro* though they disappeared from the blood when atoxyl was injected into the living animal. In atoxyl arsenic is pentavalent. Ehrlich supposed that it became actively trypanocidal in the body by being changed into trivalent arsenic. He and his colleagues investigated a long series of trivalent compounds of arsenic, which culminated in the discovery of Arsphenamine, a compound of arsenic with amino-benzene in which the arsenic is trivalent. It is an unstable compound which had to be given intravenously in a large bulk, e.g. 100 ml. or more, of sterile saline solution. It has been given in thousands of cases of syphilis with success and with few serious accidents. It did not produce blindness like atoxyl. It proved superior to mercury in syphilis especially in speed of action.

Arsphenamine was found to have a curative action not only in syphilis but in several allied diseases, e.g. framboesia (yaws) and recurrent fever.

One disadvantage of arsphenamine is its instability and the

technical difficulties of its administration. To obviate these drawbacks many related compounds have been prepared and investigated. Of these, one of the most important is *Neoarsphenamine*, B.P. In neoarsphenamine one of the NH_2 groups of arsphenamine is replaced by $NH \cdot CH_2O \cdot SONa$. Neoarsphenamine possesses certain advantages over arsphenamine which led to its superseding the latter. Especially it is more stable, does not require previous neutralization, and can be given in a smaller bulk of saline solution, e.g. 10 ml., an amount that can be given by a syringe. It is also less liable to produce toxic symptoms. The dose of neoarsphenamine intravenously is 0·15–0·6 G. It contains approximately 20 per cent. of arsenic. The maximum dose therefore contains nearly 0·12 G. of arsenic, an amount that would be fatal if given in the form of inorganic arsenic.

Among more recently introduced organic compounds of arsenic, the following may be mentioned.

Sulpharsphenamine, B.P., can be given intramuscularly or even subcutaneously when intravenous injection is contra-indicated, especially in children, 0·1–0·6 G.

One compound resembles the arsphenamines in having the As trivalent but differs in having only one benzene ring (like atoxyl). *Oxophenarsine Hydrochloride*, B.P., U.S.P., 20–60 mg., is a stable chemical substance and relatively easy to administer. It is especially useful for the intensive treatment of syphilis. This compound is given intravenously and usually distributed with buffering agents and suitable substances to render the solution physiologically compatible with blood.

It has been shown that arsphenamine and neoarsphenamine are converted in the body to oxophenarsine. The active form has thus replaced these formerly important compounds in arsenical therapy of protozoal infection.

Oxophenarsine Hydrochloride

These compounds proved of great value in the treatment of syphilis and other allied diseases. They failed, however, in two directions. They have little effect either in post-syphilitic nervous diseases such as locomotor ataxia and general paralysis, or in sleeping sickness, when the organisms have invaded the central nervous system.

Tryparsamide, B.P., U.S.P., 1–2 G., by injection, a pentavalent arsenical compound, has been used with success both in general paralysis and in sleeping sickness. One reason for the superior efficacy of tryparsamide in nervous lesions is that it penetrates into the cerebrospinal fluid better than most other arsenical compounds. Like atoxyl it is liable to produce visual disturbances, but these usually disappear when the drug is discontinued.

Toxic effects may occur after injections of the arsphenamine group of compounds. These effects may be due to the colloidal nature of the solution and come on soon after injection—symptoms, for example, such as vomiting, diarrhoea, fall of blood pressure; or anaphylactoid symptoms such as swelling of the lips and tongue, urticaria, cyanosis, and dyspnoea. More rarely, and usually at a later period, more serious symptoms may occur which are definitely a variety of arsenical poisoning; the most important of these are cerebral symptoms (*toxic encephalopathy*), jaundice which may develop into acute atrophy of the liver, and skin affections (*exfoliative dermatitis*).

The organic compounds of arsenic previously mentioned can only be given satisfactorily by injection. Other such compounds *Acetarsol*, B.P., *Carbarsone*, B.P., U.S.P., can, however, be given by mouth and have been so tried in the cure of amoebic dysentery as a supplement to emetine (p. 301). A usual dosage is 0·25 G. They are of doubtful efficacy and may prove toxic. They have been used by topical application in powder or pessary form for the treatment of leucorrhoea due to infestation of the vagina with *Trichomonas*, with variable success.

VII

DRUGS ACTING ON THE CENTRAL NERVOUS SYSTEM: *STIMULANTS*

THE cells of the central nervous system differ in structure, function, and evolution. It is therefore *a priori* unlikely that a drug will act on all nerve cells quantitatively alike, and experimentally it is found that different nerve cells vary very much in their sensitiveness to the action of drugs. Some drugs, e.g. the general anaesthetics, depress all nerve cells more or less in the same way though in differing degrees, and display only a slight degree of selective action. For as yet unexplained reasons, some drugs influence the activities of the spinal cord rather than of the cerebrum, while with other drugs the reverse is true. Some show a very high degree of selective action within the central nervous system itself; for example, apomorphine in small doses singles out the vomiting centre almost to the exclusion of other nerve cells. Moreover, a drug may depress some cells of the nervous system while stimulating others; for example, morphine may stimulate the cardiac vagus centre at the same moment as it depresses the respiratory centre.

The explanation, even the description, of the action of drugs on the central nervous system is therefore difficult, for we have not as yet even tentative explanations of their selective actions. There is no order of attack which is common to all drugs. Their effects have been determined by observation and experiment, but are arbitrary in so far as any reason can at present be given for their site and quality of action.

In accordance with the plan uniformly adopted in this book, the stimulants of the central nervous system will be considered before the depressants.

CAFFEINE

Caffeine is an active principle found in several plants which have come to be used in different parts of the world as stimulant beverages, e.g. tea in Asia, coffee and kola in Africa, maté in South America, and others. The effect originally attributed to these beverages, namely a sense of refreshment and wakefulness with a relief from fatigue and hunger, is borne out, as will presently be shown, by the pharmacological actions of caffeine. In view of the absence of any striking subjective sensations produced by these beverages, it is remarkable not only that these plants have been singled out in different parts of the world, but that no other plants containing considerable quantities of caffeine have been discovered by modern methods. Time and unaided observation seem to have been adequate for the discrimination of those plants which contain caffeine. Caffeine was first isolated over a century ago from coffee, and its identity with the alkaloid in tea shown later (1838).

ACTION ON THE CENTRAL NERVOUS SYSTEM. As is not unusual with drugs which act on the central nervous system, the action of caffeine differs somewhat in different species of animals. In all, however, the primary effect is one of stimulation. In animals with a poorly developed cerebrum, like the frog, the symptoms produced by caffeine are attributable mainly to stimulation of the spinal cord; but in mammals, and especially in man, caffeine stimulates the central nervous system in the preferential order of brain, medulla, and spinal cord. The account here given will refer to the effects of caffeine on man.

Small doses of caffeine stimulate the psychical areas of the brain. Evidence of this is seen in the increased speed and clearness of thought, in the more rapid association of ideas, and in the capacity for more prolonged intellectual effort. The feeling of mental weariness, if present, is relieved; and, as this feeling is associated with the desire for sleep, wakefulness is produced. Rather larger doses are required to stimulate the medullary centres, but, especially when these centres are depressed, the stimulant action of caffeine upon them may be pronounced.

ACTION ON THE CIRCULATION. The action of caffeine upon the circulation is somewhat complicated. In regard to both heart and vessels there are two opposing factors: the central stimulation of the vagus centre tends to slow the heart, whereas the peripheral action tends to quicken the heart; the central stimulation of the vasomotor centre tends to contract the arterioles, the peripheral action tends to dilate them. The net effect of caffeine on the circulation is therefore apt to be variable. In man the heart beats are usually quickened without any marked increase in force of beat. In regard to the purely vascular effects, it must be remembered that vasoconstrictor nerves are feebly developed or absent in the heart, lungs, and central nervous system. When, therefore, the vasomotor centre is stimulated, there is little or no contraction of the arterioles of these organs. In them the peripheral depressant action of caffeine on plain muscle is not antagonized by central stimulation. Caffeine, therefore, contracts the blood vessels of the splanchnic area, but dilates those of the heart, lungs, and brain. While there may be little change in the systemic blood pressure, there is a redistribution of the circulation, giving a better blood supply to the vital organs.

ACTION ON THE KIDNEYS. Caffeine is a diuretic, a commonly observed effect of caffeine-containing beverages. This effect is due partly to an improvement in the blood supply of the kidneys, the vessels of which are dilated while the splanchnic vessels are constricted. The blood flow through the kidneys is increased without any reduction in the pressure. There may be also an increase in the number of glomeruli functioning at any one time. In addition to these glomerular effects, reabsorption from the tubules is diminished (p. 24).

ACTION ON VOLUNTARY MUSCLES. The capacity of isolated voluntary muscle to perform work is increased by certain concentrations of caffeine. It is uncertain whether this action takes place in man with ordinary doses, but it may be a factor in explaining the relief of physical fatigue and the capacity for increased muscular effort which caffeine undoubtedly produces. This effect is, however, mainly due to the stimulation of the nerve cells, for it is these which experience fatigue before the muscles themselves are exhausted.

THERAPEUTIC USES OF CAFFEINE. The stimulant properties of tea and coffee are due to the caffeine they contain, and caffeine is of far greater importance from its general use as a stimulant in such beverages than from its purely medicinal use.

Caffeine is used as a stimulant in cases of depression of the central nervous system, for example in cases of narcotic poisoning. It is occasionally used to stimulate the respiratory and vasomotor centres in other conditions. As a diuretic, it has largely been supplanted by other xanthine derivatives.

It can be given by mouth as the alkaloid itself *Caffeine*, B.P., U.S.P., 0·3–0·6 G. (5–10 gr.). *Caffeine and Sodium Benzoate*, U.S.P., 500 mg., a mixture which is more soluble than caffeine itself, can be given by mouth or by injection.

Caffeine

$$H_3C \cdot N - C = O$$
$$O = C \quad C - N \cdot CH_3 \ (b)$$
$$H_3C \cdot N - C - N \!\!>\!\! CH$$

(*a*)

is a purine derivative, trimethylxanthine, being related, therefore, to the xanthine bodies found in the urine and tissues of animals. In the body caffeine loses its methyl groups and is excreted in the urine for the most part as dimethylxanthines and monomethylxanthines. Of the three possible dimethylxanthines, two are of medicinal importance.

Theobromine, in which the methyl group at (*a*) is replaced by H, occurs in cocoa. It has little or no stimulant action on the central nervous system which explains the absence of this action from cocoa; it is, however, a more powerful diuretic than caffeine. It is therefore preferable to caffeine for use as a diuretic because diuresis can be evoked without any undesired action on the nervous system. Theobromine is very insoluble in water but is rendered freely soluble by admixture with certain sodium salts. The B.P. has **Theobromine and Sodium Salicylate**, which is freely soluble and is used as a diuretic in doses of 0·6–1·2 G. (10–20 gr.).

Theophylline, B.P., U.S.P., in which the methyl group (b) in caffeine is replaced by H, is isomeric with theobromine. It is the most powerful diuretic of the three (60–200 mg. (1–3 gr.)).

Aminophylline, B.P., U.S.P., in which Theophylline is combined with Ethylenediamine can be given by mouth, 0·1–0·5 G. (1½–8 gr.), as tablets or in similar doses by intramuscular or slow intravenous injection. It is of value in cases of congestive heart failure and angina, acting presumably by dilating the coronary vessels, and in status asthmaticus where the beneficial effect is probably due to relaxation of the bronchial muscles.

Other Cerebral Stimulants

From the point of its general use in beverages as well as its medicinal use, caffeine is by far the most important cerebral stimulant. Many other substances are known which stimulate the brain, but none of them resemble caffeine in producing an unmixed stimulation of the higher centres. Thus cocaine (p. 133) stimulates both sensory and motor areas, and the stimulation is often followed by depression. Atropine (p. 160) stimulates rather the motor areas, and the same is true of camphor (p. 245) and absinthe. These substances have other more important actions from the therapeutic point of view, so that they are discussed elsewhere.

MEDULLARY STIMULANTS

Caffeine may be taken as a typical cerebral stimulant and strychnine as a typical spinal stimulant. Both stimulate also the medullary centres, but certain substances act principally on the medullary and hypothalamic centres and are used to stimulate failing breathing or circulation. Their clinical efficacy is doubtful in many cases and they are being used less. They have been grouped under the title of Analeptics.

Picrotoxin, B.P., a glucoside obtained from seeds of species of *Anamirta*, is in toxic doses a convulsant poison, the convulsions in mammals differing from those produced by strychnine in being of a clonic type, thus indicating an action on the higher parts of the central nervous system rather than on the spinal cord. Stimulation of the medulla is shown by quickened respiration, slowed pulse, and sometimes vomiting. It has been used especially as a stimulant in narcotic poisoning, e.g. by barbiturates. Comatose patients may tolerate relatively high doses and suitable dosage has usually to be found by trial in individual patients. A usual initial dose is 1–3 mg. intravenously, which may have to be frequently repeated and very large total doses have been given successfully.

Lobeline, an alkaloid from lobelia possessing the general actions of nicotine, is also used as a respiratory stimulant, especially in asphyxia of new-born children. It stimulates the chemoreceptors in the carotid sinus which react to an increase in CO_2, or particularly to a decrease in O_2 in the blood.

Leptazol, B.P., *Pentylenetetrazol*, U.S.P., is a white, crystalline substance, soluble in water. It is absorbed quickly from oral or subcutaneous injection. It resembles camphor in action but is more dependable. Large doses produce epileptiform convulsions, and it has been extensively used in convulsive doses in the treatment of mental disorders, especially schizophrenia, until superseded by the more readily controlled electroconvulsion therapy or the more beneficial insulin-induced coma. Smaller doses are used as a stimulant to the vasomotor and respiratory centres in cardiovascular and respiratory failure. It has an awakening effect in animals depressed by narcotics, an action sometimes termed 'analeptic', though this word is now often used to include also stimulation of the respiratory or circulatory systems.

Leptazol can be given by mouth in doses of 50–100 mg.; for parenteral injection, a 10 per cent. solution, i.e. *Injection of*

Leptazol, B.P., can be used in doses of 0·5–1 ml. as an analeptic or in much larger doses as a convulsant.

Nikethamide, B.P., U.S.P., (Coramine), is the diethylamide of pyridine-carboxylic acid, a yellow oily liquid, miscible with water. It acts generally like leptazol. It is used therapeutically only as a circulatory and respiratory stimulant, but being more slowly absorbed has a more prolonged but less powerful action than leptazol. It is given by parenteral injection in doses of 0·25–1 G. (1–4 ml. of the official *Injection of Nikethamide*). Other stimulants discussed elsewhere are nalorphine (p. 121) and amphetamine (p. 173).

STRYCHNINE

The seeds of *Strychnos nux-vomica*, a tree indigenous to south Asia, have for centuries been known to be poisonous. In the seventeenth century they were used in England chiefly as a poison for superfluous domestic animals. With the discovery, over a century ago, of the active principles of the seeds (alkaloids, strychnine and brucine), knowledge became more precise in regard to their physiological actions, and gradually strychnine attained a position of importance as a therapeutic agent, a position which it has now largely lost. Brucine acts qualitatively like strychnine, only is much weaker.

ACTIONS OF STRYCHNINE. The most characteristic and important action of strychnine is to render the reflex centres in the central nervous system more sensitive to afferent stimuli. As its main action is on the lower and more primitive part of the central nervous system—on the reflex centres—the effects produced by it are very similar in all vertebrates, whereas drugs which act on the cerebral cortex may produce very dissimilar effects in different species of vertebrates. In medicinal doses strychnine stimulates the spinal cord but not the brain, caffeine stimulates the brain but not the cord: both alkaloids have a less pronounced effect on the medullary centres.

Small doses of strychnine such as may be used therapeutically, do not alter the path of a reflex: they merely exaggerate the normal response. Larger doses cause reflex impulses to spread through the central nervous system with increasing facility, so that the normal responses may be altered. An afferent impulse, which would normally be reflected through one set of motor neurons, may now induce an ever-widening discharge of motor impulses until, with poisonous doses of strychnine, generalized convulsive movements of voluntary muscle are produced.

Owing to the nature of their production, strychnine convulsions often display a typical character. When a muscle contracts, its antagonistic muscle is not inhibited; all voluntary muscles contract more or less simultaneously, and the stronger overcome the weaker. Thus, for example, the more powerful extensor muscles of the back overcome the flexors, so that in strychnine convulsions the vertebral column may be arched with the concavity backwards—so-called opisthotonos. Convulsions are usually succeeded by intervals of complete relaxation of muscles, until the nervous system recovers from exhaustion, whereupon convulsions recur. Consciousness is retained during the convulsions, and intense pain is felt from the violent contracting or stretching of muscles. Death occurs usually from spasmodic fixation of the respiratory muscles or from exhaustion of the central nervous system, especially the respiratory centre. Strychnine convulsions are singular in the ease with which they are provoked by slight afferent stimuli, e.g. a current of air or a sudden noise.

Apart from a stimulant action on reflex centres, strychnine has no important action in medicinal doses. It temporarily increases the acuity of the special senses especially of sight, leading to an increase in the field, and in the acuity, of vision.

THERAPEUTIC USES OF STRYCHNINE. Strychnine can be used wherever it is desirable to increase reflex excitability. It is sometimes used as a respiratory and circulatory stimulant from its action on the medullary centres. It has no direct action on the heart muscle.

Strychnine Hydrochloride, B.P., is a soluble salt given by mouth or hypodermically in doses of 2–8 mg. ($\frac{1}{30}$–$\frac{1}{8}$ gr.). The *Solution of Strychnine Hydrochloride*, B.P., (1 per cent.) 0·2–0·8 ml. (3–12 min.) is a convenient form in which to prescribe it in mixtures. *Tincture of Nux Vomica*, B.P., 0·6–2 ml. (10–30 min.), made from the seeds, is still prescribed as a bitter or general tonic, but this usage has greatly declined.

VIII

DRUGS ACTING ON THE CENTRAL NERVOUS SYSTEM: *DEPRESSANTS I*

THE ALCOHOLS

ALCOHOL is of medicinal importance from several points of view. It is widely used as a solvent for the active principles of drugs. It is in common use as an external application, chiefly as an antiseptic. When taken internally its actions have a twofold interest, as a basis for possible therapeutic uses of alcohol, and as an explanation, justification, or condemnation of the use of alcoholic beverages.

ETHYL ALCOHOL

Of the series of alcohols, ethyl alcohol is from these points of view by far the most important, and therefore will be considered first.

LOCAL ACTIONS. Strong alcohol applied to the skin is irritating, especially if evaporation be prevented. It partly precipitates proteins and tends to harden the skin, and is used for this purpose to prevent bed-sores in people who are confined to bed with exhausting illnesses. It is a valuable antiseptic for the skin, especially in preparing the skin for operation. It is important to remember that the antiseptic activity of alcohol is not proportional to its concentration. The optimum concentration for antiseptic action is about 70 per cent. Both above and below that concentration it becomes less antiseptic. To a mucous membrane it is, as one would anticipate, more irritant than to the skin. In concentration it has a burning taste and irritates the mouth and alimentary canal, and continued use of strong alcoholic beverages tends to produce chronic gastritis. In concentrations below about 20 per cent., alcohol stimulates the gastric secretions.

ABSORPTION AND FATE OF ALCOHOL. This naturally depends to some extent upon the initial dilution of alcohol, upon the absolute amount of it and its relation to food, so that the following statements represent rather an average of truth. Alcohol is rapidly and completely absorbed from the stomach and small intestine. It is one of the very few substances to be absorbed from the stomach. It begins to appear in the blood in a very few minutes, and attains a maximum concentration there in from 1 to 2 hours. It disappears from the blood with surprising slowness, not completely even in 18 hours. Its disappearance is due almost entirely to oxidation of it in the tissues to acetaldehyde, only small quantities of it appearing in the urine and breath. On account of the slow rate of its oxidation, the ultimate maximum concentration of it in the blood is nearly the same when a quantity of alcohol is taken in divided doses (so long as the interval is not more than 2 hours) as when it is taken in one dose, though of course the attainment of that maximum takes longer. A given quantity of alcohol is absorbed more slowly and attains a lower maximum when taken in a dilute solution than when taken more concentrated.

ALCOHOL AS A FOOD. The oxidation of alcohol must yield energy from conversion of acetaldehyde to acetate and its utilization in the cycle of carbohydrate metabolism, and alcohol is therefore a 'food', but there are some important differences between it and other foods. In the first place the rate of alcoholic combustion, and therefore the equivalent liberation of energy, is almost independent of the concentration in the blood. About 10 ml. of absolute alcohol per hour can be oxidized by an adult man, but not more, however high the concentration in the blood. Within the limits of this rate of combustion it can replace carbohydrates and fats, and supply about one-third of the total energy requirements of the body. In the second place (unless when present in low concentrations in the tissues), it does not undergo combustion at a more rapid rate during exercise than during rest. The liberation of energy derived from its combustion is therefore not adjustable to the energy requirements of the body. Lastly, if more is taken than can be oxidized, the concentration rises in the blood, and the toxic actions of alcohol make themselves manifest.

Besides being an expensive food, it is therefore a food which is difficult to regulate and which can fulfil only a limited function. It provides no vitamins. It has one merit. It is rapidly absorbed without requiring any digestion, and, if sufficiently diluted, does not interfere with the organs or processes of digestion.

ACTION ON THE CIRCULATION. Alcohol, usually in the form of whisky or brandy, i.e. fairly concentrated, is often used as a stimulant in fainting or acute circulatory failure. Since little (or, as most people think, no) stimulation of the heart is produced when alcohol is perfused through an isolated heart, its main effect here seems to be a reflex stimulation of the circulation produced by the irritation of the mouth and stomach. Even moderate doses of alcohol produce a dilatation of skin vessels, a very general effect of hypnotic drugs.

Owing to this effect, as well as from its depressing the central nervous system, alcohol tends to lower the body temperature.

ACTION ON THE CENTRAL NERVOUS SYSTEM. By far the most important action of alcohol is its action on the nervous system. It is this action which is mainly responsible for the use and abuse of alcoholic beverages, and which has led to the prolonged dispute as to the advisability of their prohibition. Into the minor details of this action it is impossible to enter here. It is now generally conceded by those who have carefully studied the subject that alcohol is a depressant of the central nervous system, and that only under very exceptional circumstances can it be said to have any stimulant action at all. This is true whatever the dose or dilution of it.

The depressant action of alcohol is exerted chiefly on the brain, and first affects those regions or functions of the brain which are evolutionally the last to be developed. They involve those mental qualities which especially distinguish man from the lower animals, and the adult man from the child; the faculties of judgement, concentration, self-criticism, the power of 'calculating the odds', the faculty of speech, and the ability to maintain steady progression in the erect posture. As the result of depression of the higher centres, the influence of which on the lower centres is largely of an inhibitory or controlling nature, a person becomes, under the influence of alcohol, more child-like, more emotional, more reflex. Alcohol tends to induce a feeling of well-being and of freedom from care, and a subjective sensation of increased mental and physical capacity. This effect is largely due to the depression of the higher centres, with the consequent subjection of the sense of responsibility and of self-criticism. For, where mental processes or physical capacity are capable of measurement, they are found to be not enhanced but deteriorated by alcohol. A great variety of such experiments have been made, e.g. on reflex time; on association; on work involving concentration and co-ordination of muscles, such as shooting; on work involving memory, attention, and skilled muscular movements, such as typing; on endurance in marching, and so on—all of which have led to the general conclusion that alcohol lessens the acuity of mental processes and retards the execution of skilled movements.

Very large doses of alcohol depress the whole central nervous system, eventually producing paralysis of reflexes and coma, and, if the dose be fatal, death mainly from paralysis of the respiratory centre. In these doses it resembles in its effects the general anaesthetics.

TOXIC EFFECTS. These usually begin to appear at a level of 150–200 mg. alcohol per 100 ml. blood. The psychic phenomena come first and motor incoordination is usually not noticed until levels of 300 mg. per cent. or more are reached. Over 500 mg. per cent. endangers life; coma is profound and may prove fatal, particularly if inhalation of vomit should occur. Levels in recently secreted urine are somewhat lower than those in the blood but give an indication of minimum blood levels. Alcohol in the breath can be detected by simple qualitative tests.

Acute alcoholism in those not addicted to it may be treated

by washing out the stomach and giving slow intravenous injection of nikethamide (p. 82). Amphetamine is also of value. Acute alcoholism in the chronic alcoholic is better treated by administration of massive doses of vitamins by injection. This is often effective in terminating a dangerous coma. Chronic alcoholism may bring about deterioration of any organ, but the liver, the heart, and the brain are most often affected. The deterioration of mental function (psychosis) may be punctuated by episodes of acute delusional insanity (delirium tremens). These are best treated with massive vitamin therapy, withdrawal of alcohol and administration of sedatives.

Mention must be made of an interesting experiment in the prevention of alcoholism. The substance *Disulfiram*, (Antabuse) interrupts the metabolic degradation of alcohol at the stage acetaldehyde to acetate. If, therefore, this drug is administered prophylactically to the alcoholic as an adjuvant to medical and psychiatric treatment, surreptitious indulgence is quickly followed by the toxic effects of excess aldehyde in the blood—flush, headache, and burning sensations. Disulfiram has proved rather toxic and is now less widely used than at first.

Therapeutic uses of Alcohol

In an attempt to estimate the therapeutic value of alcohol, it is impossible to be brief without being dogmatic. Alcohol has so long been used in the form of alcoholic beverages, as well as for medicinal purposes, that the whole question is obscured by traditional beliefs. It is convenient to take the therapeutic uses in the order in which the pharmacological actions have been considered.

As a Stimulant of Digestion. It is a general belief that the use of an alcoholic beverage may, under certain circumstances, be an aid to digestion. The belief is well founded. This effect is due to three factors, the relative prominence of which varies in different individuals and under different circumstances. There is, firstly, the psychical effect on appetite and digestion.

If a glass of beer or of wine appeals to the palate, it will reflexly stimulate appetite and digestion. Secondly, when alcohol enters the stomach it may directly stimulate the gastric glands. This is more likely to happen if the alcohol be above 10 per cent., e.g. of the strength of wines rather than of beers (below 4 per cent.). In the third place, the depressant action of alcohol on the brain, which tends to produce a sense of freedom from care, may improve appetite and digestion in cases where anxiety or mental abstraction is likely to interfere with digestion. On the other hand, it is equally true that persons of normal health of mind and body do not require any such artificial stimulus to digestion. In cases of ill health, however, especially when accompanied by loss of weight, this action of alcohol is often beneficial.

As A FOOD. The advantages and disadvantages of alcohol as a food have already been considered. It will be obvious that, for people in normal health and receiving a sufficient diet, alcohol is a quite unnecessary food. Indeed, the probability is that it will be deleterious, because the addition of alcohol to the diet is seldom accompanied by an equivalent diminution of other foods, so that a person who regularly uses alcohol even in moderate amounts is liable to lay down a useless, and sometimes an embarrassing, amount of fat. During some acute diseases, however, and during convalescence, the mere food-value of alcohol may be considerable. It ought to be given in small quantities frequently repeated, so as to allow of its being oxidized sufficiently completely to prevent an intoxicant concentration in the blood.

As a STIMULANT TO THE CIRCULATION. As already pointed out, alcohol has no direct effect on the contractions of the heart, comparable, for example, to that of adrenaline or of digitalis. The reflex stimulation which it produces resembles rather that which can be provoked by other irritants of the mouth and stomach, and the effect is neither powerful nor lasting. Moderate doses of alcohol have little effect on the blood pressure. The dilatation of the skin vessels which it produces gives rise to a feeling of warmth, a sensation which is dependent mainly upon the blood supply to the skin. This has led to the use of alcohol in preventing the effects of 'chill'. Chill seems to be due not so much to mere exposure as to unequal exposure of the surface of the body to cold. Alcohol tends to produce a more equal distribution of blood in the skin, and does in certain circumstances prevent the effects of chill. But as the result of the dilatation of the superficial vessels, as well as from its depressant action on the nervous system, alcohol tends to lower the *body temperature*. The advisability of the use of alcohol in preventing chill will depend, therefore, upon a variety of circumstances; e.g. the age and robustness of the person, the intensity and duration of the exposure. It is near the truth to say that, if necessary at all, alcohol should be given only after exposure, and when, in warm surroundings, its action in lowering temperature would be negligible.

As a Cerebral Sedative. Probably the majority of people who take any form of alcoholic beverage take it for its depressant action on the brain. It was doubtless this action that evoked Caliban's comment: 'For the liquor is not earthly.' If alcohol possessed all its other actions but lacked this, there would be no alcohol problem. The control over the emotions and the sometimes unnecessary control over the imagination, which are acquisitions largely of adult life, are temporarily suspended by alcohol, and therefore freer play is given to the emotional side of mind. As De Quincey conversely puts it, 'Sobriety disguises a man.' The chief attraction of alcohol is that it blunts the edge of the critical faculties, which indeed is sometimes too sharp for the ordinary affairs of life.

The sedative action of alcohol is sometimes of medicinal value in facilitating sleep. It is a safe and valuable hypnotic, for example, in young children, and a 'night-cap' is not always detrimental at the other extreme of life.

The use of alcohol is not without well-known dangers. Frequent use gives rise to a habit, which it may be difficult to interrupt. Over-indulgence is disastrous. No strength of will can prevent the physiological effects of alcohol on the tissues, or the deteriorating effect of over-indulgence on the brain cells themselves.

It may seem at first sight rather a paradox that men should have come to employ, for their relief, substances having opposite actions, as exemplified on the one hand by caffeine which stimulates the brain, and on the other hand by alcohol and opium which depress the brain. But the end achieved by members of each group is different. Caffeine, by stimulating the higher functions of the brain, produces a sense of well-being due to increased capacity for mental and physical work; alcohol or opium, by depressing these functions, produces a sense of well-being due to relief from mental or physical pain. In countries where both are available, a person may elect at one time to take a beverage containing caffeine, at another time one containing alcohol; or, of course, he may disdain the use of either or both.

OTHER ALCOHOLS

The acute toxicity of the alcohols, as determined by the minimum fatal single dose, increases with the size of the molecule, so that methyl, ethyl, propyl, butyl, and amyl alcohols show a progressive increase in toxicity. The alcohols higher than ethyl alcohol are of little medicinal importance. Methyl alcohol, however, is important from the poisonous effects it may produce when used as an adulterant of alcoholic beverages or as a solvent, &c., in the arts. While the minimum lethal dose of methyl alcohol is slightly greater than that of ethyl alcohol, the former is far more poisonous that the latter, judged from any other point of view. It is more slowly destroyed in the body, an intermediate product being formaldehyde, so that intoxication with it is more prolonged and it is more likely to be cumulative. It also may produce serious symptoms which practically never occur with ethyl alcohol. Chief among these is optic neuritis, leading to blindness. The amount required to produce this varies very much in different individuals, but as little as 10 ml. is alleged to have caused blindness. The adulteration of a beverage with methyl alcohol, therefore, constitutes a very serious danger. The volatility of methyl alcohol constitutes a hazard in industry.

GENERAL ANAESTHETICS

It is interesting to remember that the applied use of general anaesthetics began not much over a hundred years ago. Forty years earlier Davy had noticed that inhalation of nitrous oxide produced a loss of sensation of pain and had suggested that it might be used for this purpose in surgical operations, but it was left for Wells, an American dentist, to rediscover and apply this action of nitrous oxide to the induction of general anaesthesia in 1844.

Long seems to have been the first to use ether as a general anaesthetic two years before, and Simpson the first similarly to employ chloroform five years later. Those three general anaesthetics were therefore all launched upon an expectant world in the space of five years, 1842 to 1847; and though some attempts were made to oppose their introduction (on the grounds that the abolition of pain was an interference with the prerogative of God), the practice of general anaesthesia rapidly spread.

Though in the original quest for a suitable general anaesthetic the discovery and adoption of volatile substances which could be administered by inhalation were largely a matter of accident, experience soon revealed certain great advantages attaching to inhalation, as compared with other methods of administration, for this purpose. The lung has a very large surface, specially adapted for rapid absorption and elimination of gases. When a volatile substance is given by inhalation, its physiological action can therefore be produced rapidly; the amount given is under continuous control; if an excessive amount has been given, further administration of the anaesthetic can easily be stopped, and, provided that circulation and respiration continue, the anaesthetic is rapidly eliminated by the lungs when its administration is discontinued. Though general anaesthesia can be produced by oral, rectal, subcutaneous, or intravenous administration of suitable substances, the maintenance of anaesthesia at an optimum level is more difficult to ensure, and, if an excessive dose be given, elimination of this excess is less easy and less rapid.

The development of modern anaesthesia has led to the clear realization that a 'general anaesthetic' has three functions to perform: (1) hypnosis—to put the patient into a light controllable coma so that he is not disturbed by the surgical procedure; (2) analgesia—to render him free from sensations of pain from manipulation of the part (local analgesia) or the whole (general analgesia) of his body; and (3) relaxation—to diminish or abolish reflex tightening of muscles which follows upon stimulation of parts and which renders surgery difficult. These effects must not endanger life and must be under control. Formerly these three essentials were combined by a general depression of all nervous function by such means as heavy dosage with chloroform or barbiturate. Now these functions are considered separately and the purpose is served by the administration of separate drugs, e.g. a 'sleep' dose of thiopentone, analgesia with inhaled nitrous oxide–ether mixture and injections of pethidine (p. 120) intravenously, and relaxation with gallamine triethiodide or curare (p. 147). At the same time the anaesthetist controls respiration and blood volume (p. 28) and subsequently ensures immediate recovery by using, as may be necessary, antidotes to the drugs administered. He is also interested in pre-operative sedation and post-operative relief of pain and may be called upon to control blood flow by administering ganglion blocking agents (p. 153) or to reduce temperature by administering chlorpromazine, &c. (p. 110), in special cases.

INHALATION ANAESTHETICS

ETHER

Ether is a colourless, mobile liquid, having a characteristic odour and a burning taste. It is highly volatile and inflammable; specific gravity about 0·7; boiling-point about 35° C.; soluble in about twelve parts its volume of water at 25° C. It is an oxide of the alkyl radical ethyl, its formula being $(C_2H_5)_2O$; and is therefore closely related chemically to ethyl alcohol, C_2H_5OH. Corresponding with this similarity in chemical constitution, ether and ethyl alcohol resemble one another also in their pharmacological actions. The differences in their action and uses, though these are of great practical importance, are due very largely to differences in their physical properties. Ether is, for instance, much more volatile than ethyl alcohol; so much so that it can be given by inhalation, because a sufficient concentration in air can be obtained to produce rapidly the full physiological actions of it. This is not possible with alcohol. Another important difference between the two is that, whereas alcohol is almost completely destroyed in the body, ether is eliminated by the lungs—very little, if any, of it being oxidized.

When given by mouth, ether can produce a kind of intoxication which is very similar to alcoholic intoxication, but its great medicinal importance rests upon its use as a general anaesthetic when given by inhalation. Like alcohol, it depresses the central nervous system, and the possibility of the employment of a substance as a general anaesthetic depends upon selective action on the central nervous system. In order that a surgical operation may be painlessly and delicately performed, not only must the sensation of pain or even consciousness be suspended, but reflex movements must also be eliminated. These conditions can be attained by paralysis of the brain and spinal cord. But a substance could not be used as a general anaesthetic if the medullary centres were simultaneously paralysed, as in that case respiratory and circulatory failure would occur at the same time as abolition of pain and reflex movement. Fortunately the vital centres are, of the whole central nervous system, least susceptible to the action of ether. Consequently the aim in giving ether as an anaesthetic is to get into the blood a sufficient concentration to suspend the functions of the brain and cord, but to stop short of that higher concentration which would paralyse the respiratory and cardiovascular centres in the medulla. This sequence of attack on the central nervous system is true of all the general anaesthetics, but it is to be remembered that it is not an inevitable sequence, because substances are known which paralyse the functions of the vital centres before those of the brain or spinal cord. General anaesthesia is produced only when ether reaches a certain concentration in the blood. Usually this takes several minutes, during which time the concentration is gradually rising, and the symptoms correspondingly changing. For convenience in comparing anaesthetics, one may consider (1) the local action of the anaesthetic, (2) the induction stage, and (3) the anaesthetic stage. Details of administration of anaesthetics can best be learnt practically. To induce anaesthesia, ether has to be inhaled in a concentration of about 6 per cent. (by volume) in air. Less is required to maintain anaesthesia once it is induced. This vapour is irritant, and may produce the usual effects of irritation of the upper air passages, e.g. salivation, coughing, increased discharge from the respiratory glands. During the induction stage, the general symptoms resemble first those of deepening alcoholic intoxication. The senses become less acute, and there is vertigo with loss of muscular control. Usually there is a period of excitement marked by tremor, struggling, or shouting, with imperfect consciousness. These symptoms are generally supposed to be due to the paralysis of the higher and inhibitory centres of the brain. As the anaesthetic is continued, depression spreads down the central nervous system, sensations, including that of pain, are abolished, the muscles relax, and eventually (after 10–30 minutes) the reflexes disappear, and the patient is unconscious and motionless apart from the movements of respiration. At this time neither respiration nor circulation is materially affected. If ether is pushed beyond this stage, the respiratory centre is paralysed, but the blood pressure is usually fairly high and the heart continues beating for some time after respiratory movements cease. If respiration does stop, artificial respiration promptly applied is usually successful in restoring normal breathing. Excessive bronchial and salivary secretion, which is one factor in predisposing to pulmonary complications, can be prevented by previous administration of atropine, which also protects the heart from vagal stimulation. The peak of the atropine effect is reached about 1 hour after subcutaneous injection.

Liability to explosions must be kept in mind, especially when ether is given with oxygen, and due precautions must be taken for absence of open flame, cautery, &c.

All volatile anaesthetics (with the possible exception of nitrous oxide) but especially chloroform, are liable to produce ketosis, due to the imperfect oxidation of fats and consequent accumulation of acid ketone compounds. Vomiting occurring during or after anaesthesia is sometimes due to this. Administration of glucose may prevent or relieve ketosis; prolonged starvation increases the risk of its occurrence.

For use as an anaesthetic ether must be of a high standard of purity and, so purified, is called *Anaesthetic Ether* (with the synonym Ether) in the B.P. and simply *Ether* in the U.S.P. For use as a solvent, &c., ether need not pass such stringent tests and such ether, which is cheaper, is called *Solvent Ether* in the B.P. and *Ethyl Oxide* in the U.S.P. Care must be taken that only the former type of Ether is used as an anaesthetic.

Ether is rarely now used by itself for induction of unconsciousness as it is too slow. It is, however, often given volatilized in Nitrous Oxide and Oxygen to deepen anaesthesia temporarily. It is of especial value in that it does not easily depress the circulation and its peripheral curare-like blocking action on the skeletal muscle motor nerve junction aids relaxation.

CHLOROFORM

Chloroform, B.P., U.S.P., $CHCl_3$, is a clear colourless mobile liquid, having a characteristic odour and a burning sweetish taste. It is soluble in about 200 parts of water; specific gravity about 1·5, boiling-point about 61° C.

Chloroform resembles ether as a general anaesthetic, but is more powerful; to produce anaesthesia, the concentration of ether in the blood has to be 3 to 6 times as high. The induction stage tends to be less prolonged, and the excitement less marked with chloroform than with ether, and the former is more pleasant to take. These differences are outweighed by the superior safety of ether, which in an equal number of administrations may cause less than one-third as many deaths. Death from chloroform may arise in three different ways.

1. Early in its administration, indeed often before the patient is anaesthetized, the heart may suddenly stop from fibrillation of the ventricles; a result of sensitization of the heart to circulating adrenaline. When the ventricles fibrillate the pumping force of the heart ceases immediately. The gravity of this condition consists in its occurring with little or no warning, and in the great difficulty of restarting the heart.

2. Death may occur at any time during the administration merely from too high a concentration in the blood. When this happens the respiration fails first, but at this time the circulation is also enfeebled.

3. Especially in patients with hepatic or renal disease, or if the liver glycogen is at a low level at the time of operation, chloroform may give rise to destructive changes in the liver. In these cases, after recovery from the anaesthetic, the patient may develop vomiting, delirium, and a rapidly fatal coma. This type of 'delayed' poisoning usually begins one or two days after anaesthesia.

NITROUS OXIDE

Nitrous Oxide, B.P., U.S.P., N_2O, is a colourless gas which for convenience of use is stored under pressure in metal cylinders, coloured blue. When pure nitrous oxide is inhaled, it rapidly produces unconsciousness, usually without any marked stage of excitement. When a mixture of air and nitrous oxide, containing anything less than 80 per cent. of the latter, is inhaled, it produces a kind of intoxication, often accompanied by laughter, whence the name 'laughing gas'; but in this case no complete anaesthesia is produced.

Nitrous oxide is not decomposed in the body, and its contained oxygen is useless for the purpose of respiration. Obviously, therefore, if it is inhaled pure, it will produce asphyxia. To be used as a general anaesthetic, it must be given in a sufficient concentration to produce general anaesthesia without producing a dangerous degree of asphyxia. This problem has been solved in two chief ways.

1. For very short operations, for example the removal of

teeth, the administration of a few inhalations of almost pure Nitrous Oxide can produce general anaesthesia. In order that the patient should receive the gas undiluted, a special apparatus is necessary, involving a mask fitting closely over the face. A device for the administration of a self-limiting supply of Nitrous Oxide during labour pains is still widely used in midwifery.

The chief advantages of this method of producing general anaesthesia are as follows: Anaesthesia is rapidly produced, and previous special preparation of the patient is not absolutely necessary. The patient can be anaesthetized in the sitting position. There are no important after effects, the patient being normal, as far as the anaesthetic is concerned, in a few minutes. Lastly, the method is the safest of all methods of producing general anaesthesia. Against these weighty advantages is the great disadvantage of the shortness of the anaesthesia, which lasts only from 20 to 60 seconds, more prolonged anaesthesia being impossible owing to the onset of asphyxia.

2. For more prolonged anaesthesia, nitrous oxide can be given (with the help of a specially designed apparatus) mixed with pure oxygen. A mixture of 90 per cent. of nitrous oxide and 10 per cent. of air will contain only 2 per cent. of oxygen. This is insufficient to prevent anoxaemia. A mixture of 90 per cent. of nitrous oxide and 10 per cent. of oxygen will, however, give a sufficiently high concentration of the former to act as an anaesthetic and enough oxygen to prevent serious anoxaemia. That nitrous oxide has a direct depressant action on the central nervous system is shown by the fact that a mixture of 90 per cent. nitrogen with 10 per cent. of oxygen has no comparable anaesthetic action.

The older general anaesthetics, ether, chloroform, and nitrous oxide have been in use for a century. From the account given of them it will be clear that none of them provides an ideal anaesthetic for all purposes. During the century the quest has continued, intensified during the last two or three decades, to discover safer and more efficient anaesthetics. The results, generally speaking, have been to discourage the idea of a 'universal' anaesthetic, which is perhaps just as improbable as a universal antiseptic, purgative, or hypnotic. There are so many variable factors involved in a surgical operation—the age of the patient, the health of individual organs (e.g. heart, lungs, and liver), the site of the operation, and the probable duration of the anaesthesia. At the present time the skilled anaesthetist needs not only knowledge of techniques but experience to decide which of the available anaesthetics is most suitable for a particular operation in a particular patient. It will be readily understood also that a method of anaesthesia which might be preferred in the operating theatre of a hospital, with all its resources of skill and apparatus, might be quite inapplicable under less advantageous domiciliary conditions.

Of the newer anaesthetics only those which have been admitted into both B.P. and U.S.P. need be mentioned here.

Ethyl Chloride, B.P., U.S.P., C_2H_5Cl, is a very volatile liquid which boils at 12° C. The vapour volatilized is inhaled by the open method or through a mask. It induces anaesthesia quickly, but prolonged anaesthesia is difficult to maintain with safety. It is chiefly used for induction of anaesthesia and for short operations.

Ethyl chloride may also be used as a local anaesthetic, for which purpose it is sprayed in a fine jet on the surface. It causes loss of sensation largely by freezing the tissues due to its rapid evaporation.

Vinyl Ether, B.P., U.S.P., $(CH_2:CH)_2O$, a liquid more volatile and less irritant than ether, is administered by open method by a mask much in the same way as ethyl chloride. Anaesthesia is produced very rapidly and there is little irritation of the respiratory tract or post-operative nausea. It is chiefly used for short operations, e.g. for dental surgery, in children, and for induction of anaesthesia, e.g. followed by ether for longer operations.

It is used for much the same purposes as ethyl chloride which it has to a considerable extent supplanted mainly because it is less likely to cause vomiting or collapse. It is highly inflammable and forms explosive mixtures with air or oxygen.

Trichloroethylene, B.P., U.S.P., CHCl:CCl$_2$, (Trilene) a colourless mobile liquid, in odour and taste resembling chloroform, was introduced as an anaesthetic in 1941. It is not irritating and induction of anaesthesia is smooth and rapid. It can be used alone or in association with nitrous oxide or ether. It is not inflammable or explosive. It has deservedly acquired a reputation for safety and is much used in midwifery, minor surgery, and dentistry. Atropine should be given previously if possible.

Cyclopropane, B.P., U.S.P., (CH$_2$)$_3$, a gas heavier than air, is a powerful anaesthetic. It is given in a concentration of 7–30 per cent., depending on the depth and duration of anaesthesia desired. The mixture is explosive and cyclopropane expensive, so that it is given by a closed-circuit apparatus both for safety and economy. Its chief advantages are the absence of irritation of the air passages and of asphyxia. It requires particularly expert administration. The cylinders are coloured orange.

NON-INHALATION ANAESTHETICS

The anaesthetics previously discussed are all sufficiently volatile to permit of their being given by inhalation, and the advantages of administration by this channel have already been mentioned. Anaesthesia can be produced also by any type of administration which secures a sufficient and safe concentration of the drug in the blood to effect the desired degree of depression of the central nervous system. Thus anaesthesia can be produced by oral, rectal, or parenteral administration. When an anaesthetic or other drug is given orally, rectally, or subcutaneously the concentration in the blood gradually rises as absorption proceeds. If the symptoms of this rising concentration show that the dose has been excessive, it is practically impossible to recall the unabsorbed portion of the drug. On the other hand, when an anaesthetic is given by inhalation the unabsorbed portion is outside the body and can be instantly removed; the concentration in the blood can also be altered from moment to moment. When an anaesthetic is given intravenously there is no unabsorbed fraction of the drug to be reckoned with; it is all thrown into the blood. In this case the actual amount put into the blood stream is known and thus effective dosage is more accurate. It would seem, therefore, that, if the dose of an anaesthetic were calculated according to body weight and it were injected intravenously, the exact degree of resultant anaesthesia could be predicted. Unfortunately this is not the case because individuals vary in their tolerance to anaesthetics at least as much as to alcohol or any other drug. This difficulty can be partially overcome by gradual intravenous injection and by employing these agents for the purpose of inducing and maintaining a moderate depth of unconsciousness and not a 'full anaesthesia'. In this way their great advantage of rapid and smooth action is retained and their dangers avoided. The practice of endotracheal intubation and controlled respiration with oxygen-enriched gas mixtures administered from a rubber bag has removed their chief danger—that of sudden arrest of breathing.

Of the barbiturates (p. 107) which have been used as anaesthetics, two deserve mention.

Thiopentone Sodium, B.P., U.S.P., introduced in 1935 is a yellowish hygroscopic powder, distributed sterile in glass ampoules. For use the powder, which is rapidly soluble, is dissolved in sterile distilled water, usually to give a concentration of 5 per cent. This solution is injected intravenously and 4 or 5 ml. may produce anaesthesia in just over half a minute. More may be administered as may be necessary for anaesthesia. It may be used either as a basal anaesthetic or as a sole anaesthetic for short operations. Anaesthesia may last for 5–10 minutes.

It is contra-indicated in hepatic disease and in asthmatic conditions—in the latter because, like many barbiturates, it is liable to produce broncho-constriction. Administration in young children may be difficult owing to restlessness and the difficulty of introducing the needle into a small vein.

Pentobarbitone Sodium, B.P., U.S.P., (Nembutal), is identical in structure with thiopentone, apart from having an O atom replacing the S atom. It can be given orally, $0 \cdot 1$–$0 \cdot 2$ G. ($1\frac{1}{2}$–3 gr.), or intravenously. It has a more prolonged action than thiopentone ($1\frac{1}{2}$–2 hours).

PREMEDICATION AND BASAL ANAESTHETICS

In recent years efforts have been made to supplement the action of general anaesthetics by drugs which act as adjuvants either in relieving pain or in suppressing muscular movements. A patient may receive, prior to the actual operation, a dose of Morphine or Pethidine, sufficient to produce drowsiness and diminution in sensitivity to pain. He will then be less upset by the unavoidable discomforts attendant upon the general anaesthetic and less of the latter will be necessary to abolish pain completely. Moreover, as the effect of morphine in reducing pain lasts for some hours, the effect will tend to endure after the anaesthetic has been eliminated. Hyoscine (p. 114) may be given with morphine to blunt the memory of the proceedings when the patient regains consciousness. Tubocurarine, gallamine, or suxamethonium (p. 150) may be administered intravenously to relax the skeletal muscles especially of the abdomen. On all such occasions controlled respiration is essential.

It has already been mentioned that a quick-acting and non-irritating volatile anaesthetic like ethyl chloride or vinyl ether can be used to induce anaesthesia which can subsequently be maintained with nitrous oxide or ether. This still involves the mechanical procedures of a volatile anaesthetic. Another method is to use some form of 'premedication' in which a supplementary depressant can be administered by another channel. The hypodermic use of morphine has been mentioned. One or other of the barbiturate group (p. 107) can be given in doses to produce effects ranging from simple sedation to narcosis. For example, a patient can be rendered unconscious in seconds by an intravenous injection of Thiopentone, following which anaesthesia can be continued by Nitrous Oxide and Ether.

If the depressant produces a degree of anaesthesia which persists during the period of administration of the volatile anaesthetic, it can be regarded as a 'basal anaesthetic' (e.g. bromethol) and it enables an equal depth of anaesthesia to be attained with a lower concentration, and smaller total amount, of the volatile anaesthetic.

Bromethol, B.P., *Tribromoethanol Solution,* U.S.P., (a solution of Tribromoethyl Alcohol in Amylene Hydrate), also known as Avertin, was introduced about 30 years ago as a hypnotic and general anaesthetic. For the latter use it has been given up owing to difficulty of dosage. It is still used as a basal anaesthetic. It is given by rectum and the dose has to be calculated to body weight. Induction is pleasant and irritation of the respiratory tract is avoided. Amnesia for the period of the operation usually occurs. It is slowly excreted. It has also been used as a sedative in mania, status epilepticus, and tetanus.

IX

DRUGS ACTING ON THE CENTRAL NERVOUS SYSTEM: *DEPRESSANTS II*

HYPNOTICS

As has already been pointed out, chloroform produces, at the commencement of induction of general anaesthesia, a condition of drowsiness, due to depression of the higher centres of the brain. At this stage there is no marked impairment of motility or alleviation of pain. Chloroform might be used therefore merely for the induction of sleep in people suffering from insomnia. It would, however, be difficult and even dangerous to administer for this purpose, and, moreover, its action would be too evanescent. Merely for inducing sleep it would clearly be an advantage to have a substance which could be given by mouth and which would produce a slighter but more enduring effect. About twenty years after the introduction of chloroform anaesthesia, Liebreich discovered (1868) that a substance, chloral hydrate, possessed these properties, and it was the first of a long series of compounds to be tried for use as hypnotics, only a few of which can be mentioned here.

Prior to the discovery of the hypnotic action of chloral, only such naturally occurring substances as opium had been used to produce sleep. The members of the group first to be considered are often called artificial hypnotics, because they are manufactured in the laboratory, in contradistinction to such substances as opium which are derived from plants. The words hypnotic, soporific, and narcotic are all used to designate drugs employed to induce sleep.

CHLORAL

Chloral Hydrate, B.P., U.S.P., $CCl_3 \cdot CH(OH)_2$, is a chlorinated derivative of ethyl alcohol. It is a colourless, crystalline substance, freely soluble in water, with a burning taste and pungent fruity odour.

It has an irritant action and consequently it must be given well diluted, otherwise it may cause vomiting. Owing to its solubility it is rapidly absorbed when given by mouth, and exercises its main action on the central nervous system, which it depresses. Given by mouth in a dose of 1 G. (15 gr.), it produces within half an hour a condition of drowsiness which, under favourable conditions, will induce sleep. This sleep is hardly distinguishable from natural sleep and usually passes off in 6 to 8 hours, by which time most of the chloral has been excreted.

If the dose be increased, e.g. 3 G. (45 gr.), the sleep produced is deeper, the patient more difficult to arouse, and the sensation of pain is dulled; the respiration is slower, and the pulse may be weaker. With still larger doses, complete anaesthesia with abolition of reflexes is produced—a condition almost identical with chloroform anaesthesia. It would be difficult to use it as a general anaesthetic in man, however, because the anaesthetic dose is too near to the dose which also paralyses the respiratory centre.

Chloral depresses the central nervous system very much in the same order as the general anaesthetics; that is, first the brain, then the spinal cord, and lastly the medullary centres. Medicinal doses stop short of the last action, and produce a dulling of the activities of the brain and spinal cord. It is used therapeutically in cases of insomnia and nervous excitability.

In large doses chloral depresses the heart muscle as well as the respiratory and vasomotor centres, but there is no danger of this happening with medicinal doses. Chloral is therefore an excellent and reliable hypnotic.

In the body it is mostly reduced to trichlorethyl alcohol which combines with glycuronic acid, and the resulting combination, called urochloralic acid, together with some unchanged chloral, is excreted in the urine.

Chlorbutol, B.P., *Chlorobutanol*, U.S.P., forms colourless crystals, resembling camphor somewhat in odour and taste and soluble 1 in 125 of water. It acts as a hypnotic like chloral and is also a local anaesthetic and antiseptic. It is used as a gastric sedative, e.g. in sea-sickness, where it exerts a local anaesthetic action on the stomach as well as a central sedative action after absorption (0·3–1·2 G. (5–20 gr.), in cachets or as a suspension).

Paraldehyde, B.P., U.S.P., $(CH_3 \cdot COH)_3$, a polymer of acet-aldehyde, bears a considerable resemblance chemically to chloral but contains no chlorine. It is a mobile liquid, soluble 1 in 10 of water; with a hot, burning taste and persistent, unpleasant odour. It was introduced as a hypnotic in 1882. It acts very like chloral, and produces sleep in about 15 minutes. Its chief advantage is its safety and that, owing to its disagreeable taste and smell, it is less liable than other hypnotics to induce habit formation, though this may occur. Its chief disadvantage is that it is disagreeable to take and, owing to its slight solubility, rather difficult to dispense elegantly. The usual dose is: B.P., 2–8 ml. (30–120 min.); U.S.P., 4 ml. It may be injected or prescribed in iced water, brandy and water, or in capsules.

Paraldehyde is also used, mostly by rectal administration, as a basal anaesthetic in children, one advantage claimed for it being the absence of respiratory depression.

Carbromal, a ureide containing bromine, is a mild hypnotic and sedative, given in doses of 0·3–1·0 G. (5–15 gr.). It acts promptly and has a shorter action than chloral hydrate. It is comparatively safe and free from unpleasant effects. It may be combined with a barbiturate.

BARBITURATES

Barbitone was introduced as a hypnotic in 1903. It is diethyl-barbituric acid, barbituric acid being a compound of urea and malonic acid.

$$2 \ CO \begin{matrix} \nearrow NH—CO \searrow \\ \\ \searrow NH—CO \nearrow \end{matrix} C \begin{matrix} \nearrow C_2H_5 \\ \\ \searrow C_2H_5 \end{matrix}$$

Since its introduction a large number of allied compounds have been investigated and over a score of them have come into therapeutic use. It will be possible here to mention only a few of the more widely used compounds. The generic termination 'one' is used in B.P. names, 'al' in U.S.P. names, e.g. barbitone is identical with barbital. Apart from this a particular compound may have more than one trade name which often leads to confusion.

Usually new compounds are formed by substitution at points **4**, **5**, and **2** on the graphic formula.

SUBSTITUTION AT **4**. Acidic compounds like barbitone are usually very insoluble in water but they form monosodium derivatives (e.g. sodium barbitone) that are freely soluble, —NH—CO—C— in the ring changing to —N═CONa—C—. For injections such salts must be used and they may also act more rapidly when given by mouth. The character of the action is unchanged.

SUBSTITUTION AT **5**. Substitution of one or sometimes both ethyl groups by alkyl or other groups of varying length, e.g. phenobarbitone, has produced a large number of compounds, differing chiefly in speed and duration of action.

SUBSTITUTION AT **2**. Replacement of the O atom by S produces thiobarbiturates which usually have a brief powerful action, e.g. thiopentone.

Barbiturates differ mainly in duration of action due to differences in the rate of excretion by the kidney and of destruction by the liver and also to the extent of storage in body fat, but they also differ to some extent in the site and intensity of their actions on the central nervous system. This allows them to be used for different conditions, ranging from simple hypnosis to more profound sedative actions.

Barbiturates which are used mainly as simple hypnotics will, in continuance of the previous drugs in this chapter, be first considered. The drug to be preferred will depend on the type of insomnia. The hypnotic action should coincide with the expected time of wakefulness, though this is less easy as there are wide variations in response. If a patient has difficulty in getting off to sleep a quick short-lasting hypnotic is indicated. If the patient wakes in the middle of the night and is then unable to get to sleep, a hypnotic with a more delayed and lasting action, if given at bedtime, will be preferable.

Among those with a quick and short action are **Quinalbarbitone Sodium**, B.P., **Secobarbital Sodium**, U.S.P., (Seconal Sodium). It acts in 15–20 minutes, lasts for 3–6 hours, and is comparatively safe given in doses of 50–200 mg. ($\frac{3}{4}$–3 gr.). Cyclobarbitone (Phanodorm), 200–400 mg. (3–6 gr.) is very similar.

With a rather longer action (4–8 hours) are Butobarbitone (Soneryl) and **Pentobarbitone Sodium**, B.P., (Nembutal), both given in doses of 0·1–0·2 G. ($1\frac{1}{2}$–3 gr.).

Among long-acting barbiturates (8–16 hours) are **Barbitone Sodium**, B.P., 0·3–0·6 G. (5–10 gr.) and **Phenobarbitone**, B.P., U.S.P., 30–120 mg. ($\frac{1}{2}$–2 gr.). In small doses they are useful in maintaining mild sedation but hypnotic doses tend to make the patient drowsy next morning, which has led to their less frequent use for this purpose. Phenobarbitone has a special action in diminishing motor overactivity (p. 112).

Hepatitis and nephritis are a contra-indication to the use of long-acting barbiturates. Overdoses cause especially depression of respiration and coma, which is often prolonged and, with a fatal dose, always precedes death.

Repeated and continuous use of barbiturates for insomnia may lead to a degree of habituation that makes sleep difficult without them and may provoke restlessness and mental upset if they are suddenly discontinued. They are prescribed too recklessly and often without due supervision. They have become suicidal poisons. Cases of acute poisoning should be treated by gastric lavage, stimulants such as picrotoxin, amphetamine, or bemegride, with oxygen therapy if needed. In prolonged coma, penicillin may be given in an attempt to forestall hypostatic pneumonia. Chronic poisoning with barbital is characterized by impaired mental acuity, diplopia, ataxia, occasionally cyanosis, and an erythematous rash.

SEDATIVES

Recently much attention has been given to a search for substances which could relieve mental anxiety and stress without impairing cerebration or producing depression or drowsiness. Such drugs are sometimes referred to by the seductive name of 'tranquillizers'. Their permanent value in therapeutics is not still precisely established. It can be expected that their indiscriminate use will not be without hazard.

Chlorpromazine Hydrochloride, U.S.P., dose: oral 100 mg. daily; intramuscular and intravenous 25 mg. daily, is related structurally to the antihistamine promethazine (p. 183) and has a very complicated set of actions including depression of the vomiting centre and of the heat-regulating centre, intensification of the action of hypnotics, analgesics, and local anaesthetics, and peripheral actions on the autonomic system. It has been used to produce 'hypothermia' as an adjunct to anaesthesia in surgical operations. As a sedative it has been used for reducing states of excitement. Cases of anxiety neurosis experience a relief of tension and a feeling of well-being. It may also be prescribed for nausea and vomiting, vertigo and motion sickness. Side-effects which may arise from chlorpromazine include dryness of the mouth, disturbances of bladder or bowel action, pyrexia and skin eruptions. More serious are jaundice and, rarely, agranulocytosis.

Reserpine. When Extracts of *Rauwolfia serpentina* (p. 154) were used as hypotensive agents, it was noticed that they relieved neurotic symptoms in hypertensive patients. This is mainly due to an alkaloid reserpine, which seems to act on the subcortical regions of the brain. It has been used as a cerebral sedative, but opinions as to its value are rather conflicting.

Methylpentynol. This is an unsaturated tertiary alcohol, soluble about 1 in 10 in water. It has a sedative action and sufficient doses (0·5–1 G.) may induce sleep. It is used to relieve minor phobias and for premedication in children, e.g. before tonsillectomy or dental attention. It may also be helpful in asthma and as a sedative in aged patients in whom barbiturates may increase mental confusion and restlessness.

ANTICONVULSANTS

In a number of diseases an explosive overactivity of the motor area of the cerebral cortex may occur, resulting in disorderly contractions of skeletal muscles. If these spasms are intermittent and jerking in nature the convulsion is called 'clonic'; if they are sustained for longer periods without intervening relaxation it is called 'tonic'. Convulsions may occur as an incident in many diseases, particularly in febrile disorders in young children, but the commonest cause is the condition of idiopathic epilepsy. This disease may be classified roughly into three clinical groups which it is important to distinguish in order to select the appropriate drugs for treatment:

(i) *Grand mal*, the classical 'fit', in which there are loss of consciousness, clonic and tonic spasms, frequently incontinence of urine and faeces, followed by stupor;

(ii) *Petit mal*, characterized by fleeting blunting or loss of consciousness with often only momentary interruption of what the patient was doing or saying. In more severe attacks the patient may fall down and there may be slight convulsive movements of the face or arms;

(iii) *Psycho-motor epilepsy*, characterized by loss of memory or self-consciousness and automatic or irresponsible behaviour which may have serious social consequences. In most cases of epilepsy, abnormalities of the electro-encephalogram can be detected.

BROMIDES. Among simple salts, bromides occupy a peculiar position owing to their depressant action on the central nervous system, due to the bromine ion and produced by every compound which liberates it in the blood. Bromides are rapidly absorbed from the intestine and distributed and excreted exactly like chlorides. The kidney does not differentiate between them but excretes them in the urine in the same proportions as they occur in the blood. If a single dose of bromide is given, some of it therefore appears quickly in the urine but it may take weeks before the last traces are eliminated. Consequently bromides accumulate in the blood if given continuously. As a result of this, undesirable effects ('bromism') may occur, of which the most usual are disturbances of digestion, skin eruptions, and mental impairment.

Bromides in sufficient doses induce symptoms of impaired mental activity, lethargy, diminished reflex excitability, and drowsiness. Pain sensation is hardly affected, but the excitability of the motor cortex is reduced. Very large doses produce incoordination of movement and stupor. The chief action of bromides is therefore to diminish the excitability of the motor areas of the brain.

Bromides were for long the only effective remedy for epilepsy. They usually reduced the number of fits in grand mal, but, when given over long periods, were liable to produce bromism. Bromides are sometimes used for insomnia due to worry, often combined with chloral hydrate, but they have now been largely replaced by newer remedies. The official salts are *Potassium Bromide*, B.P., and *Sodium Bromide*, B.P., U.S.P., 0·3–1·2 G. (5–20 gr.).

Phenobarbitone, B.P., *Phenobarbital*, U.S.P., is similar to barbitone, but that one ethyl group is replaced by a phenyl group, whence its official name. It is a white powder, soluble only 1 in 1,000 in cold water. It has a more prolonged action than barbitone, and is more valuable for subduing motor excitability. Though it can still be used as a sedative and hypnotic (p. 109), it has found a special place in the treatment of epilepsy, in which it is usually superior to bromides in reducing the number of fits. In epileptics medication may have to be continued for years and chronic toxicity may occur with phenobarbitone. The soluble *Phenobarbitone Sodium*, B.P., is often given intramuscularly for convulsive disorders in children. The oral dose of Phenobarbitone is 30–120 mg. ($\frac{1}{2}$–2 gr.).

Phenytoin Sodium, B.P., *Diphenylhydantoin Sodium*, U.S.P. This compound which contains the five-membered ring of hydantoin in place of the six-membered ring of the barbiturates, was introduced in 1938 as a remedy for convulsive disorders. In the treatment of epilepsy it is often superior to phenobarbitone in controlling the fits and in producing more frequent and longer remissions. A variety of toxic side-actions have been observed, e.g. skin eruptions, pyrexia, gingivitis, diplopia, and ataxia. The B.P. dose is 50–100 mg. ($\frac{3}{4}$–1$\frac{1}{2}$ gr.).

Methoin, B.P., (Mesontoin), 50–100 mg., is a compound related to phenytoin with similar actions. Gradual increase of dosage is recommended because a few patients get allergic skin rashes. Otherwise it seems devoid of many of the side-effects of phenytoin, while having a good effect in controlling epilepsy.

Primidone, B.P., has been tried with success in patients resistant to other drug therapy. The optimum daily dosage is 1–1·5 G. in divided doses. With all anticonvulsant drugs the minimum effective dosage for each patient has to be approached by graded increases of a low initial dosage. Particular care has to be taken while substituting one drug for another. Primidone is not very toxic.

All these compounds are of little value in petit mal but in 1945 there was introduced *Troxidone*, B.P., *Trimethadione*, U.S.P., which in doses of 1–2 G. daily is effective in helping many sufferers from this complaint. The immediate side-effects of taking this compound, as with all cerebral depressants, may be a variable amount of dizziness and drowsiness but in addition it may produce a form of 'dazzle' or photophobia, skin rashes, and depression of the blood-forming organs.

DRUGS USED IN THE TREATMENT OF PARKINSONISM

Paralysis agitans, first described by Parkinson in 1817, is a degenerative disorder of the extrapyramidal system evidencing itself usually in middle or late life. A symptomatically similar condition often follows encephalitis lethargica, a virus disease which spread rapidly over the world in epidemic waves from 1917 to 1925. The name Parkinsonism is applied to the syndrome exhibited in both these diseases. The chief symptoms are: difficulty with certain muscular movements especially with the finer and more skilled movements of the fingers (often first attracting attention by a deterioration of handwriting); disorder of movements of the internal and external muscles of the eyes; rigidity of the muscles, sometimes accompanied by tremor, and excessive salivation.

Hyoscine Hydrobromide, B.P., *Scopolamine Hydrobromide*, U.S.P. For long this condition was treated with large doses of Extract of Belladonna (p. 160) which contains the alkaloids Atropine and Hyoscine. It is the latter which exerts the depressant effect on the so-called hyperkinetic state by affecting the basal ganglia, the reticulum of the brain-stem and the associated nuclei through which motor impulses and reflex patterns are modified. Hyoscine relieves the rigidity of the muscles but not the tremor: salivation is reduced by the peripheral depressing action at the nerve-ends.

Synthetic antihistamine compounds such as *Promethazine Hydrochloride*, B.P., and *Diphenhydramine Hydrochloride*, U.S.P., (Chap. XIV), are of some value.

Ethopropazine is related in structure to them, and may relax the stiffness and occasionally diminish tremor in Parkinsonism. It is a central depressant which exerts a degree of peripheral atropine-like activity. It may cause dizziness, dryness of the mouth, and some blurring of vision. The dosage of Ethopropazine is 0·3–0·4 G. per day.

Caramiphen has similar properties and similar drawbacks which include gastric irritation. Readily absorbed and quickly destroyed it shows no signs of chronic toxicity.

Benzhexol is a cortical stimulant, countering the apathy and lethargy which is a feature of many cases of Parkinsonism. The dosage is 5–10 mg. per day. None of these drugs is curative; after interruption of treatment the symptoms recur.

Mephenesin has little effect on the higher centres but depresses spinal reflex centres and may help to relieve spasm associated with such conditions as disseminated sclerosis. It is an antidote to strychnine poisoning, when it may be given with care by intravenous injection.

DRUGS USED FOR MOTION SICKNESS

The nausea and vomiting from which many people suffer when travelling by boat, car, train, or aeroplane may make travel a misery. The causation is complicated, labyrinthine disturbance being perhaps the chief factor, aggravated by obscure sensations from the gastro-intestinal tract, by unaccustomed smells, or even by suggestion. Only in recent years have systematic attempts been made to assess the relative values of the many remedies proposed, old and new.

Hyoscine Hydrobromide, by its sedative central action and its peripheral action on the alimentary canal can, in doses of 0.5–1 mg. generally be relied on to check motion sickness. Several antihistamines (p. 182) have been found effective, e.g. Promethazine, which has a short action, and Diphenhydramine, which has a prolonged action. The latter compound combined with chlorotheophylline goes under the name Dimenhydrinate. It can be given by mouth or per rectum. The antihistamines may cause drowsiness or fatigue in some people. Central depressants such as phenobarbitone and chlorbutol seem, from recent experiments, less effective.

X

DRUGS ACTING ON THE CENTRAL NERVOUS SYSTEM: *DEPRESSANTS III*

OPIUM ALKALOIDS

OPIUM is the dried juice obtained from the unripe capsules of the white poppy, *Papaver somniferum*, which is cultivated chiefly in south Asia. It has been used as a narcotic from very early times. It surpasses all known drugs in relieving pain in doses which do not conspicuously impair other functions of the brain, and this property, together with others only less important, makes it one of the most valuable of remedies.

Opium owes its pharmacological actions to the alkaloids contained in it, of which there are many. The most important of these is morphine, which forms about 10 per cent. of opium. Morphine was first isolated from opium in 1814, and has gradually supplanted opium for many purposes. Morphine has the advantages over opium that it has an unvarying composition and, in the form of a salt, can be injected hypodermically. The actions of opium are due mainly to morphine, but the presence of other alkaloids which do not act precisely like morphine makes the actions of opium not identical with those of morphine. The alkaloids occurring in opium fall structurally into two distinct groups: (1) derivatives of phenanthrene, (2) derivatives of isoquinoline. To the former belongs morphine. The morphine molecule possesses two OH groups, one phenolic, the other alcoholic. In codeine the phenolic hydroxyl is replaced by a methoxyl group. Of the isoquinoline alkaloids the most important is papaverine.

MORPHINE

Morphine, though acting mainly as a depressant, does not affect the functions of the central nervous system quite in the same way as the general anaesthetics and hypnotics, but displays a more marked selective action than they do. The medicinal dose of morphine is 8–20 mg. ($\frac{1}{8}$–$\frac{1}{3}$ gr.). The smaller of these doses produces a feeling of drowsiness with disinclination for movement, a distinct lessening of the sensation of pain if present, and some slowing of the respiration. If the environmental conditions are conducive to it the patient may pass into a light sleep. In a dose of 15–20 mg. ($\frac{1}{4}$–$\frac{1}{3}$ gr.) morphine produces deeper sleep from which the patient can be temporarily aroused. The respiration is distinctly slower, the skin somewhat congested and the pupils are contracted. With still larger doses the pupils become still smaller, coma deepens, and, in fatal cases, death occurs from arrest of respiration.

These symptoms point to a depression of the central nervous system beginning with the higher centres. The loss of judgement, combined with exaltation of imagination and relief of pain and discomfort, is largely responsible for the pleasure which some people derive from morphine and for the seductive habit which it may create in them.

THERAPEUTIC USES. The chief therapeutic value of morphine depends upon its power to relieve pain, physical discomfort, and mental anxiety. A dose which will relieve pain may leave intelligence but little impaired. A constant pain is relieved better than sudden sharp pain. It has therefore a wide use for the relief of pain, sleeplessness due to pain, or restlessness and anxiety due to haemorrhage, &c. Owing to the serious danger of habit-formation, it is specially indicated only in acute disease of short duration or in pain of terminal diseases.

It is of no value in the treatment of conditions of excessive *motor* excitability, e.g. in epilepsy or in strychnine poisoning.

Morphine depresses the cough centre. It is widely used for this action in checking useless cough (i.e. cough which is not fulfilling its physiological function of clearing the air passages) when that is interfering seriously with the well-being or sleep of the patient.

Morphine is also used for the relief of severe colic and abdominal pain. It effects this partly by its central analgesic action, but in some conditions it also quietens intestinal movements. It may also cause contraction of the pyloric and ileocolic sphincters, leading to a delay in the passage of the gastric and intestinal contents. It therefore tends to produce constipation, and is sometimes used in the treatment of diarrhoea.

Morphine is excreted partly by the kidney and partly by the mucous membrane of the alimentary canal. When it is taken habitually a high degree of tolerance may be acquired to it, so much so that an *habitué* may take with impunity quantities which would kill several people unaccustomed to it. Various reasons have been given to explain this tolerance, e.g. increased destruction of the alkaloid in the body or more complete elimination, but, in addition to this, the cells of the central nervous system become less sensitive to it.

Codeine resembles morphine in action, but is weaker and less certain. It is chiefly used in the form of *Codeine Phosphate*, B.P., U.S.P., 10–60 mg. (⅙–1 gr.) in the treatment of cough, or as *Tablets of Codeine Phosphate*, B.P., or *Compound Tablets of Codeine*, B.P. (containing also Aspirin and Phenacetin), for relief of arthritis or myalgic pains or for headaches. It has the merit of rarely inducing habit-formation.

Papaverine Hydrochloride, B.P., U.S.P., differs from morphine in chemical constitution and to some extent in pharmacological action. It has a feebler depressant action on the central nervous system and tends to relax smooth muscle; whereas morphine, in some animals at least, stimulates smooth muscle. It is chiefly used in angina pectoris, bronchial asthma, and in renal and biliary colic, for its effect in relaxing smooth muscle; B.P., 0·12–0·25 G. (2–4 gr.) orally; U.S.P., 30 mg. by injection.

Opium, being a mixture of these alkaloids, acts in the main like morphine, but, owing to its content of the isoquinoline alkaloids, it may have a depressant action on smooth muscle unlike pure morphine. Artificial mixtures of opium alkaloids, e.g. papaveretum, act like opium, and can be given by hypodermic injection, whereas preparations of opium are given by mouth.

Preparations of Morphine and Opium

Like other alkaloids morphine itself is insoluble in water, but its salts are soluble in varying degrees, so that morphine is usually prescribed in the form of one of its soluble salts, e.g. *Morphine Hydrochloride*, B.P., U.S.P., soluble in 23 parts of cold water 8–20 mg. ($\frac{1}{8}$–$\frac{1}{3}$ gr.). A salt of morphine can be prescribed as required, but, for convenience, the B.P. contains a *Solution of Morphine Hydrochloride* 1 per cent., 0·3–2 ml. (5–30 min.) for oral administration. *Morphine Sulphate*, B.P., U.S.P., soluble 1 in 21, is official in both pharmacopoeias (U.S.P., average dose 15 mg.), and both have also an official *Injection of Morphine Sulphate* for hypodermic use.

Powdered Opium, B.P., U.S.P., may be given in doses of 30–200 mg. ($\frac{1}{2}$–3 gr.), or in the form of one of its numerous preparations. Of these only two may be mentioned. *Tincture of Opium*, B.P., (Laudanum), containing 1 per cent. of morphine, is given in doses of 0·3–2 ml. (5–30 min.) B.P.: 0·6 ml. U.S.P. Where a weaker preparation is desired, e.g. in the treatment of cough or diarrhoea, *Camphorated Tincture of Opium*, B.P., which contains opium and aromatic substances, may be given in doses of 2–4 ml. (30–60 min.). Children, especially infants, are very intolerant of morphine or opium.

SYNTHETIC MORPHINE-LIKE COMPOUNDS

The opium alkaloids hitherto discussed are alkaloids which occur naturally in opium and can be extracted from it. Other alkaloids have been artificially prepared from morphine, of which three may be mentioned.

Diamorphine (Heroin) is a diacetylmorphine, which very closely resembles morphine in action and has been widely used as a substitute for morphine. It is more powerful and has a smaller dose.

It is very liable to give rise to a habit which is even more difficult to stop than the morphine habit. It is less liable than morphine to produce constipation. Owing to its liability to produce habit, it is no longer official.

Dihydromorphinone Hydrochloride, U.S.P., (Dilaudid), 2 mg., is closely related chemically and pharmacologically to morphine and is chiefly used for the relief of pain and cough. It is less liable than morphine to produce nausea or constipation. Like morphine it can produce euphoria, addiction, and tolerance.

Ethylmorphine Hydrochloride, U.S.P., is not used as an analgesic, owing to its local irritant action, but this action is utilized in cases of corneal ulcer in which the local application of a solution (5–10 per cent.) produces a vasodilatation which has a favourable effect on the condition.

Many synthetic compounds less closely related to morphine have been investigated with a view to discovering analgesics equal to morphine in efficiency but free from its dangers.

Pethidine Hydrochloride, B.P., *Meperidine Hydrochloride*, U.S.P., a piperidine compound much simpler than morphine in structure, was introduced in 1939. It has the central analgesic action of morphine, but the relief of pain is generally not so pronounced or so lasting. It has also a relaxing effect on smooth muscle (somewhat resembling papaverine) which has led to its use in conditions of spasmodic contraction of such muscle, e.g. in asthma and various kinds of colic. It depresses the medullary centres less than morphine and hence is less useful for cough but possibly preferable as a pre-anaesthetic analgesic (p. 103). It is also a local anaesthetic and has a quinidine-like action on heart muscle. It is given either by mouth, by subcutaneous or intramuscular injection, 25–100 mg., or by intravenous injection, 25–50 mg.

As an analgesic it is a satisfactory substitute for morphine in many conditions. It has been especially recommended in labour. It is relatively free from toxic effects; sweating, dizziness, and more rarely vomiting are the most common side-actions. Tolerance and addiction may result from repeated use but less commonly than with morphine

Methadone Hydrochloride, B.P., U.S.P., (Amidone), has, in similar doses, a slightly greater analgesic action than morphine but little or no sedative action. It is especially useful for relieving pain without producing mental dullness. It is readily absorbed when given by mouth and, in doses of 5–10 mg. in tablet form, may obviate the need for injections of morphine. Like morphine it depresses the respiratory and cough centres and often controls cough in small doses. It does not cause spasm of smooth muscle. It is liable to cause addiction and tolerance. Among the side-actions that may occur are dizziness, dry mouth, and sweating.

Among other less popular synthetic substitutes for morphine may be mentioned *Phenadoxone Hydrochloride*, B.P., 25–50 mg. by mouth, 5–15 mg. by subcutaneous or intramuscular injection.

Two derivatives of morphine have quite different actions from the parent alkaloid but may be conveniently discussed here, though they are not used as analgesics.

Nalorphine, N-allylnormorphine, proved an ineffective analgesic but was found to antagonize the C.N.S. depression produced by morphine and related alkaloids, such as diamorphine, pethidine, and methadone. It does not antagonize barbiturates. It may act partly by competition for the appropriate receptors in the central nervous system. It is not a direct stimulant apart from poisoning cases. In morphine addicts it may precipitate severe withdrawal symptoms. It is used as the *Injection of Nalorphine Hydrobromide*, B.P., containing 10 mg. in 1 ml., *Nalorphine Hydrochloride Injection*, U.S.P., 5 mg. in 1 ml., and it is given intravenously in doses of 5–10 mg., repeated if necessary, in poisoning due to morphine and similar narcotics.

In obstetrics it is sometimes used in doses of 0·1–1 mg. injected directly into the umbilical vein of the new-born child for respiratory failure resulting from administration of narcotics to the mother during labour.

Apomorphine is an artificial derivative of morphine formed from the latter by the action of certain dehydrating agents whereby it loses a molecule of water. This chemical exchange entails a considerable change in physiological action, for in apomorphine the depressant action on the central nervous system is greatly enfeebled, while the stimulant action on some medullary centres, which is displayed to some extent by morphine in certain animals, is enormously enhanced. This is especially shown on the vomiting centre. In small doses apomorphine has little action beyond inducing vomiting and the usual concomitants of vomiting, e.g. increased bronchial and sweat secretion. Unlike most emetics (e.g. copper sulphate and ipecacuanha) it acts directly on the vomiting centre and thus can advantageously be given hypodermically. It acts very rapidly—within a few minutes—and is used in cases of poisoning to empty the stomach: *Apomorphine Hydrochloride*, B.P., 2–8 mg. ($\frac{1}{32}-\frac{1}{8}$ gr.), U.S.P., 5 mg. hypodermically as an emetic.

INDIAN HEMP

The hemp plant, *Cannabis sativa*, has been used for centuries in Asia and Africa for its intoxicant or narcotic action, acting in some ways like opium.

The effects vary in different persons, but a dreamy condition with lack of restraint and loss of appreciation of time and space are common. Preparations of hemp go under many names, Haschish, Bhang, Banja, Marihuana, &c.

It gives rise to a habit, prolonged indulgence in which may predispose to mania or other nervous disorders. It has been used medicinally to induce sleep, but is uncertain in action, partly from its poor keeping qualities. It is no longer official.

ANTIPYRETICS AND ANALGESICS

Phenol, as well as many of its allies, lowers the temperature of the body if given in large doses. Some of them, e.g. phenol and creosote, have been used medicinally for this purpose, but have been found too dangerous for general use as antipyretics.

In 1875 it was discovered that salicylic acid lowers the temperature in some fevers. Before that time the chief antipyretic known was quinine. Quinine, as will be seen presently, has some antipyretic action under any conditions, but a very marked action in malaria. In this disease, however, the reduction in temperature is due mainly to destruction by quinine of the causal organism of the disease, and the improvement or cure of the condition is due to the destruction of the parasite and not to the lowering of the temperature. This association of an antipyretic and curative action in quinine is accidental. The antipyretics to be discussed in this chapter do not usually, so far as is known, kill off the organisms which are provocative agents of fever. While experience has shown that there is no sound reason for routine interference with a moderate pyrexia, yet often the mere reduction of fever may diminish the discomfort of the patient and tend to produce sleep. Moreover, it has been found that nearly all the antipyretics have also an analgesic action; they relieve pain by an action on the central nervous system. While, therefore, antipyretics as a class are not definitely curative agents, they have important uses: (1) for the reduction of fever which is so high as to be, *per se*, dangerous, (2) for the reduction of moderate pyrexia in certain conditions, and (3) for the relief of certain kinds of pain.

SALICYLATES AND RELATED COMPOUNDS

Salicylic Acid, B.P., U.S.P., differs from phenol in having a carboxyl group in the ortho-position, which renders it much less toxic than phenol. Its two isomers meta- and para-oxybenzoic acids have neither the therapeutic nor the toxic actions of salicylic acid. Salicylic acid forms fine, colourless, needle-shaped crystals, soluble only about 1 in 500 of water. Sodium salicylate is freely soluble in water.

Salicylic acid is an irritant to all tissues, and causes some pain and irritation of the stomach when swallowed. It has a nauseous, sweet taste. It is a good antiseptic and is chiefly used in skin diseases, e.g. in the form of the *Ointment of Salicylic Acid*,

B.P., (2 per cent.). Salts like sodium salicylate have a much feebler antiseptic action.

It is absorbed rapidly from the intestine, and circulates in the blood in the form of sodium salicylate. The actions of salicylic acid and of sodium salicylate after absorption are therefore identical. Salicylic acid and its salts are important chiefly for their action in rheumatic fever. In this fever salicylates lower the temperature, and also relieve the pain of the inflammatory joint lesions. The antipyretic action of salicylates resembles that of the more regular antipyretics of the phenacetin group, that is to say it is an action on the heat-regulating centre, increasing heat-loss by dilatation of the skin blood vessels and by profuse sweating. It is difficult to explain the beneficial action of salicylates in rheumatic fever solely by this antipyretic and analgesic action, because no other antipyretics or analgesics have an equally potent effect in this particular disease, and conversely salicylates are not equally antipyretic in fevers other than acute rheumatism. It cannot be a very powerful action, because the duration of the disease is not materially shortened nor is the danger of the spread of the lesion, e.g. to the valves of the heart, markedly lessened by salicylate treatment. In this treatment of rheumatic fever dosage is important. Relatively large initial doses are required to relieve the pain and fever, after which the continuance of this relief can be maintained by smaller doses. These may have to be continued for weeks before the fever permanently subsides; otherwise the symptoms may recur when salicylates are discontinued. A common practice is to begin with a dose of 4 G. (60 gr.), followed by 1·2 G. (20 gr.) every two or three hours until the pain or fever is subdued, after which the dose may be lessened, e.g. to 4 G. (60 gr.) in 24 hours. The effect is, of course, due to the salicyl ion in the blood, and it is from that point of view immaterial whether it be given in the form of salicylic acid or of sodium salicylate.

Sodium Salicylate, B.P., U.S.P., is preferable, (1) because it is far less irritant to the stomach, and (2) because it is more easily prescribed owing to its easy solubility. The hydrochloric acid of the stomach will free the salicylic acid from sodium salicylate, and to check this, as well as to promote excretion, it is usual to prescribe with it an alkaline salt like sodium bicarbonate. Ordinary doses of salicylates have usually no important effects beyond those described, but large doses in all people, and ordinary doses in people who are specially susceptible to their action, produce characteristic symptoms, of which the chief are headache, nausea, vomiting, tinnitus, deafness, and vertigo, and sometimes skin rashes and albuminuria. These symptoms of 'salicism' have a superficial resemblance to the symptoms of cinchonism (p. 297). Salicylic acid is excreted in most secretions but chiefly in the urine, in which it occurs partly combined with glycuronic acid. Excretion begins in about 15 minutes and goes on for one or more days according to the dosage.

Other salicyl compounds have been introduced into medicinal use, of which the following may be mentioned.

Methyl Salicylate, B.P., U.S.P., or Oil of Wintergreen, is a colourless liquid, chiefly used for local application to the skin over rheumatoid painful areas like lumbago.

Acetylsalicylic Acid or Aspirin, B.P., U.S.P., 0·3–1 G. (5–15 gr.) is a white powder sparingly soluble in water, almost tasteless, and less irritating to the stomach than salicylic acid. Part
of it is split up in the intestine into acetic and salicylic acids, but some of it is absorbed as the unchanged molecule. While generally its actions after absorption are similar to those of sodium salicylate, the fraction that is absorbed unchanged alters the action, especially in two ways. In the first place, aspirin is a more general analgesic than sodium salicylate, and is very commonly used to relieve headaches and the pains of non-articular rheumatism. In the second place, the toxic symptoms produced by it are rather different. It is rare for therapeutic doses of it to induce untoward symptoms, but in a few

persons it may produce faintness, cyanosis, oedema of the face, or asthma. Aspirin is often compounded with other analgesics such as codeine or phenacetin, or diaphoretics such as ipecacuanha. The danger of local concentrations of released salicylic acid eroding the stomach may be avoided by using *Soluble Tablets of Acetylsalicylic Acid*, B.P., which are readily disintegrated in water before consumption. That the primary pharmacological action of aspirin is that of a depressant of the central nervous system is readily seen in the effects of overdosage. Moderate amounts cause flushing, sweating, overbreathing, and salicism; larger doses produce a profound and often fatal coma. Treatment is with gastric lavage, alkali by mouth and intravenous infusion of glucose and sodium bicarbonate or Ringer-Lactate Solution (p. 27).

Benzoic Acid, B.P., U.S.P., $C_6H_5 \cdot COOH$, owing to the absence of a hydroxyl group, is physiologically less active than salicylic acid, but resembles it qualitatively. It has a feeble action in acute rheumatism. It is a less powerful antiseptic than salicylic acid, and is chiefly important from its use to prevent or delay bacterial decomposition in preserved foods or beverages. *Benzoin*, B.P., U.S.P., an oleo-resin obtained from *Styrax benzoin*, contains benzoic acid and has been used as an antiseptic. *Compound Tincture of Benzoin*, B.P., (Friars' Balsam) is used in expectorant mixtures, and has also been used as an antiseptic for boils, abrasions, &c. Benzoic acid is excreted in the urine in combination with glycine forming hippuric acid, the synthesis taking place in the kidney.

DERIVATIVES OF ANILINE: ANTIPYRETICS OF THE PHENACETIN GROUP

While antipyretic and analgesic actions, obscurely present in phenol, are conspicuous in salicylic acid and its near relatives, these actions are even more pronounced in certain derivatives of aniline. Aniline has some antipyretic action, but produces dangerous collapse and destruction of red blood cells. It is oxidized in the body to para-aminophenol. By the entrance of an acetyl group into the molecule, the aniline is rendered less toxic and more resistant to oxidation. The resulting substance, acetanilide, has been used as an antipyretic and analgesic, but toxic effects with it were common.

Phenacetin, B.P., 0·3–0·6 G. (5–10 gr.), *Acetophenetidin*, U.S.P., 300 mg., in which an ethoxyl group has been introduced into acetanilide, has replaced it.
It is now believed that the anti-
pyretic and analgestic action both of acetanilide and of phena-cetin is due to the formation in the body of N-acetyl-*p*-amino-phenol, $C_6H_4 \cdot OH \cdot NH \cdot CO \cdot CH_3$. If this substance is formed rapidly, temperature falls too quickly and rises again too soon, and also toxic actions are more likely to occur, because the con-centration of N-acetyl-*p*-aminophenol in the blood is higher for a time. With phenacetin the formation of N-acetyl-*p*-aminophenol occurs more slowly than with acetanilide and its effects are correspondingly less drastic and less transient. Phenacetin has been used in numberless cases both as an antipyretic and as an analgesic, and, with medicinal doses of it, toxic effects are almost unknown.

Numerous derivatives of aniline have been investigated and many of them found to have antipyretic and analgesic actions like phenacetin, but none of them are superior to it in safety and efficiency. Phenazone (antipyrin) had a long vogue as an antipyretic and analgesic but idiosyncrasy to it, with collapse and cyanosis, was fairly common and it is now rarely used. Amidopyrine has also been discarded owing to its liability to produce agranulocytosis.

Agranulocytosis is a disorder recognized since 1922 and characterized by sore throat, fever, and prostration with ex-treme reduction, or almost total absence, of granulocytes in the blood. It is always a serious, and sometimes a fatal, condi-tion. Amidopyrine was found to be a common cause of it but many other drugs have been incriminated, among them some sulphonamides, thiouracil, gold, isoniazid, and phenylbutazone.

As other allergic symptoms, e.g. urticaria or asthma, may be associated with it, it has been suggested that it may be some kind of allergy.

Phenylbutazone, B.P., (Butazolidin), 0·2–0·4 G. daily in divided doses, acts as an analgesic and antipyretic in a similar way to those compounds discussed above and to which it is chemically related. It has been recommended especially for pains of rheumatoid arthritis which it often promptly relieves. A variety of toxic reactions may occur from it, including skin rashes, haemorrhages, peptic ulcer, vomiting, and jaundice. The most serious complication is however agranulocytosis, of which there have been a number of fatal cases. It should not be given without adequate control, and some investigations have shown that, in relieving arthritic pains, it is not definitely superior to sufficient doses of aspirin, which is much safer.

METHOD OF ACTION OF ANTIPYRETICS. The heat-regulating centre in the brain maintains the body temperature constant within fine limits by balancing heat-loss against heat-production. But this balance is often upset in disease, especially by the action of bacterial toxins. These usually raise the body temperature to a level which is characteristic for the particular toxin producing the fever. The antipyretics which we have previously considered, and of which the most important are sodium salicylate, aspirin, and phenacetin, all lower a febrile temperature by increasing heat-loss, through dilatation of the skin vessels and increased sweating. Those effects are not due to a peripheral action of those substances upon the vessels and sweat-glands, but to an action on the heat-regulating centre itself. In a fever the temperature may rise to a certain level, e.g. 103° F. The heat-regulating centre is still operative, but, under the influence of the toxin, can only maintain the temperature at this higher level. The condition has often been compared to the setting of a thermostat to a higher level. The foregoing antipyretics 'set' the centre so that it maintains the temperature at a normal, or at least lower, level. The antipyretic action is therefore due to a direct selective action upon the nerve cells of the heat-regulating mechanism. It is not, so far as is known, due to a destructive action upon the bacteria causing the fever or to any neutralizing action upon their toxins.

These antipyretics have a second action. They are also *analgesics*. They relieve pain by a depressant action on the pain centre in the thalamic region, and are now more frequently used for the relief of pain than for the reduction of temperature.

They relieve pain somewhat in the same way as morphine though not so powerfully, but are for various reasons much safer than morphine. They are to be preferred to it whenever possible, but there are some cases of pain which nothing but the opium alkaloids will adequately relieve.

Antipyretics of the foregoing phenacetin group are often called 'artificial antipyretics' because they are manufactured synthetically, in contradistinction for example to quinine, which is a natural alkaloid. Quinine not only differs in structure from the members of the phenacetin group, but also offers a striking contrast to them in its method of action. For whereas the artificial antipyretics lower a febrile temperature by increasing heat-loss through their action on the heat-regulating mechanism in the central nervous system, quinine lowers the temperature (1) by diminishing heat-formation through an action on the tissue-cells, and (2) in malaria, by a destructive action on the pathogenic organisms that provoke the fever. Seeing that the latter effect is by far the more important, quinine can be more appropriately considered later. Attention is merely drawn here to the existence of this other type of antipyretic (p. 296).

XI

DRUGS ACTING ON SENSORY NERVES

I. *STIMULANTS OF SENSORY NERVE-ENDINGS*

It is a very ancient and widespread practice to apply to the skin, as a remedial measure, substances which are found on investigation to have no property in common other than that of being irritants; but, though it is admitted that this practice often produces beneficial effects, there is still some doubt as to how precisely these effects are brought about. Irritation of the skin is in itself not a desirable condition, and it is now known that most of the beneficial effects produced by it are due to reflexes from the skin. As these arise from stimulation or irritation of the sensory nerve-endings in the skin, the group of skin irritants, *counter-irritants*, or *rubefacients* can conveniently be considered here.

COUNTER-IRRITANTS OR RUBEFACIENTS

When an irritant is applied to the skin, the skin becomes warmer and redder, and there may be some swelling. This is due to local dilatation of the arterioles and probably also of the capillaries, and is brought about by an axon reflex. The irritation of the skin causes an impulse to pass through the sensory nerve, which is reflected through the vasodilator nerve to the arterioles and causes them to dilate. This reflex is independent of the central nervous system and is prevented by local anaesthesia of the skin. The beneficial effects of irritants upon certain kinds of chronic inflammation of the skin and mucous membranes are mainly due to this vascular effect ('rubefacient action') accelerating repair by improving the local blood supply.

In addition to this local vascular effect irritation of the skin may produce an effect upon the general circulation, for excitation (if not too severe) of any sensory nerve stimulates the vasomotor centre and produces a reflex rise of blood pressure. The respiratory centre may also be stimulated. Many of the uses of skin irritants, such as the use of a mustard footbath in preventing the effects of chill, are no doubt due to an alteration of the blood supply brought about by a general slight rise of blood pressure added to a local dilatation of the blood vessels.

Some of the uses of skin irritants cannot, however, be explained so simply, especially the influence of irritation of particular areas of skin upon the condition of particular internal organs. In this connexion the work of Head and Mackenzie reconciled and explained some otherwise disconnected observations, examples of which will first be given in regard to one particular organ, the stomach. (1) Disease of the stomach is often associated with pain felt not in the stomach itself but over the epigastrium. (2) It had been found empirically that the application of a counter-irritant to the same area of the epigastrium relieved pain associated with gastric disease. (3) The only connexion between the stomach and the skin of the epigastrium is that the nerves of both enter the same segment of the spinal cord.

It is supposed that an afferent stimulus may, if of sufficient intensity and duration, produce a condition of heightened sensibility in the segment of the cord which it enters. Thus, in regard to (1), abnormal impulses arising from a diseased stomach and producing a condition of heightened sensibility in the corresponding segment of the cord may affect neighbouring synapses in the segment, e.g. those belonging to the sensory nerves to the skin which enter this particular segment. The irritation of the latter will be propagated to the brain and may give rise to sensations of pain, but which will be 'felt' in the skin of the epigastrium. This offers at any rate some explanation of 'referred' pain, (1) above, namely pain felt in a particular area of skin but due not to any pathological condition of the skin itself, but to a pathological condition of an internal organ.

If, under these conditions, an irritant be applied to the skin of the epigastrium, the afferent path for the stimuli arising from this point and leading to the perception area of the brain will be the same path as that of the referred pain associated with disease of the stomach. It is supposed that these new stimuli may occupy this path to the exclusion of the stimuli giving rise to referred pain, and this offers some explanation of (2), namely, how the application of an irritant to the skin of the epigastrium may relieve pain associated with disease of the stomach.

These considerations will perhaps supply some explanation of the therapeutic uses of counter-irritants. They may be useful in chronic inflammations of the skin or subcutaneous tissues— from the improvement of the local blood supply caused by the dilatation of the blood vessels. Applied to the appropriate 'Head's Areas' of the skin, they may relieve pain due to disease of the corresponding internal organs.

Many substances have been used as counter-irritants, those which have been singled out for preference being such as produce the desired amount of irritation of the skin within a reasonable time and without producing any permanent damage to the tissues. Of these may be mentioned some volatile oils (p. 243), especially *Turpentine Oil*, B.P. This can be used in the form of *Liniment of Turpentine*, B.P. *Liniment of Camphor*, B.P., (Camphorated Oil) (p. 245), acts similarly.

Mustard, which is frequently used medicinally and domestically as a rubefacient, owes its action to a volatile oil. Black mustard seeds, *Brassica nigra*, contain a glucoside and a ferment. In the presence of moisture the latter acts on the former and liberates the volatile oil of mustard. The pungency of mustard when used as a condiment and its irritant properties are due to this volatile oil. Ingested in large quantities mustard will produce vomiting, and is occasionally used as a reflex emetic. Applied to the skin, it will act as a counter-irritant.

Many other substances, apart from the volatile oils, can be used as skin irritants; e.g. alcohol, chloroform, ammonia, iodine, camphor, capsicum.

II. *DEPRESSANTS OF SENSORY NERVE-ENDINGS*

LOCAL ANAESTHETICS

COCAINE

When the Spanish conquered Peru they found that the Indians there were accustomed to chew the leaves of a shrub, *Erythroxylon coca.* 'When I asked some of these Indians why they carried these leaves in their mouths, which they do not eat, but merely hold between their teeth, they replied that it prevents them from feeling hungry, and gives them great vigour and strength.' This early account of the coca leaf was found to be no mere traveller's tale, for scientific investigation has shown that cocaine, the chief alkaloid of the leaf, has actions which explain such statements, and which are indeed its main actions; for it stimulates the central nervous system and so relieves the sense of fatigue, and, by its local anaesthetic action on the mucous membrane of the stomach, it relieves the sensation of hunger.

The stimulant properties of the coca leaf were recognized for over 300 years before the local anaesthetic action of its alkaloids was utilized. The alkaloid cocaine was isolated from the leaf in 1860 and its local anaesthetic action definitely demonstrated in 1880, when von Anrep found that, after injecting a solution of cocaine under the skin of the arm, the part became insensitive to the pricking of a needle, and that painting the tongue with a 1 per cent. solution caused loss of sensibility and of taste over the painted area. Four years later Koller showed that instillation of a solution into the eye induced sufficient anaesthesia of the conjunctiva to enable painless operations on the eye to be performed. Since then the drug has come into general use as a local anaesthetic. Before this time no efficient local anaesthetics were known, and it is difficult to realize that the current methods of local anaesthesia, which now occupy such an important place in operative surgery, are of so recent an origin.

Though of less practical importance, the actions of cocaine

on the central nervous system may be discussed before its local anaesthetic actions.

Cocaine is a powerful stimulant of the *central nervous system*, especially of the higher centres of the brain; but its action is not confined to these centres so exclusively as is the action of caffeine. Mental processes, so far as they have been measured, have been found to be temporarily facilitated by cocaine, and there is increased wakefulness and lessened sensation of fatigue, as with caffeine. But in other respects cocaine resembles atropine in its action, in stimulating motor areas as well. There is, for example, in man, restlessness, increased movement, and talkativeness; and, experimentally in animals, the motor cortex is found to be more sensitive to stimuli. With increasing doses the action spreads downwards through the central nervous axis, causing a stimulation of the medullary centres, and eventually of the spinal cord. With poisonous doses convulsions may be produced.

The stimulation of the nervous system is followed, if the dose be sufficiently large, by paralysis, affecting the centres nearly in the same sequence as the stimulation, the psychical centres being depressed first. Repeated doses of cocaine lead rapidly to the formation of a 'habit', and it is highly probable that the seductiveness of cocaine is due not entirely to the stimulant action (for no such habit is formed for caffeine) but is due partly to the depressant action on the higher centres. The latter may occur at a time when the rest of the nervous system is stimulated. In the case of acute poisoning by cocaine, the symptoms vary according to the dose and the speed of its absorption; the convulsions being sometimes so severe as to demand alleviation by chloroform, in other cases the symptoms being mainly those of paralysis. In any case, respiratory failure is usually the main cause of death, and artificial respiration is often successful in preventing a fatal issue. Especially if it should gain entrance into a vein, cocaine is also highly toxic to the heart, and in this way death may occur within a few minutes.

Cocaine has also an action on *involuntary muscle*, generally first stimulating and then depressing it. The heart is quickened and the blood vessels contracted by small doses. The constriction of the blood vessels is seen in the blanching of the conjunctiva which results from the application of cocaine to it. The pupil, on the other hand, is dilated by cocaine, whether the latter reach the pupil from local application or from the blood stream. Stimulation of sympathetic nerve-endings would explain the contraction of the vessels and dilatation of the pupil, but cocaine does not reproduce other adrenergic actions, and those two effects seem due to a specific sensitization of the muscle to adrenaline.

LOCAL ANAESTHETIC ACTION. This is the most important action of cocaine, and is due to the fact that cocaine has a specific paralysing action on sensory nerves due to its stabilizing the surface potential of the nerve fibres and so raising the threshold of excitability. It temporarily abolishes conduction in them without seriously interfering with other cells with which it may come into contact. Applied to the surface of the tongue, a solution of cocaine paralyses first the receptors of pain, then those of touch, and lastly those of taste. When applied to a nerve fibril or nerve trunk, it will abolish conduction in them. If the nerve trunk contains both afferent and efferent fibres, the former are paralysed earlier or by weaker solutions. As the cocaine is gradually absorbed into the blood, this action on the nerve passes off. Cocaine can thus be used to render a region of the body temporarily anaesthetic, so as to admit of operations being performed on that part. The difference between such local anaesthesia and general anaesthesia is that, in the former case, pain of only a limited region of the body is abolished, and, since this is due to an action on the peripheral nerves, there is no unconsciousness. A general anaesthetic acts on the central nervous system, abolishes pain over the whole body, and, in full anaesthesia, abolishes also consciousness and reflex activity.

According to the site of the afferent path to which it is applied, cocaine can produce anaesthesia of varying extents of the body. For convenience, we may consider four possible types of local anaesthesia, recognizing that these do not involve any difference in the action of cocaine but only an alteration in the site of its application. Actually cocaine itself is used in present-day practice as a surface anaesthetic, as less toxic anaesthetics have displaced it for injection purposes, so that in regard to the following uses cocaine may be taken merely as a type.

1. *Surface Anaesthesia.* When a solution of cocaine hydrochloride is applied to a mucous membrane, afferent conduction from the affected area is abolished. For example, if applied to the nasal mucous membrane, cocaine not only renders the mucous membrane insensitive to pain and touch, but also abolishes the sense of smell. A solution of cocaine does not easily penetrate the epidermis, so that it produces very little effect on unbroken skin, even if an ointment of cocaine be rubbed into the skin. These superficial actions of cocaine are due to its paralysing the afferent nerve-endings or possibly the commencing fibres of the nerve itself.

2. *Hypodermic Anaesthesia.* When cocaine is injected under the skin or mucous membrane, it comes in contact with the smaller nerve fibrils. These are readily paralysed by cocaine. A local area of anaesthesia develops, the extent of which depends upon the number of afferent fibrils which the cocaine reaches and upon the area from which they conduct sensation.

3. *Regional Anaesthesia.* The smaller nerve fibrils coming from different areas of skin join together to form larger and larger nerve trunks. If cocaine be applied to a large afferent nerve trunk it will therefore render anaesthetic a large area, the extent of which depends upon the fibrils which have their conduction abolished. Applied, for example, to the sciatic nerve, cocaine will destroy the sensibility of more or less of the corresponding lower limb.

4. *Spinal Anaesthesia.* If a cocaine solution be injected into the subdural space of the spinal cord, e.g. by passing a long injecting needle between the laminae of the lumbar vertebrae, the posterior nerve roots with which it comes into contact are

paralysed, and this abolishes sensation in their peripheral distribution. Anaesthesia of the lower limbs and of an extent of trunk depending upon the site of injection can thus be induced.

By these different methods sensation of varying regions of the body can be abolished, and painless operations done on these areas.

In the early days of its use cocaine sometimes caused serious and even fatal accidents from the poisonous effects it produced after absorption. This danger is lessened by the practice of adding to the cocaine solution a small quantity of adrenaline. The effect of adrenaline is to constrict the arterioles of the injected area, whereby it produces three salutary effects, all due to vasoconstriction, which diminishes, or for a time may even stop, the local circulation. In the first place, haemorrhage is lessened. In the second place, absorption of cocaine into the general circulation (the rate of which depends upon the efficiency of the local circulation) is slowed, so that (a) less cocaine is needed to produce anaesthesia, and (b) the anaesthesia lasts longer. In the third place, as the rate of absorption of cocaine is diminished, while the rate of its excretion is unaltered, the concentration in the blood does not reach so high a level as it would do if cocaine were injected without adrenaline, and thus the risk of general poisoning by cocaine is lessened. Even with the addition of adrenaline, cocaine is more toxic than procaine and some other local anaesthetics.

Cocaine, B.P., is generally used as *Cocaine Hydrochloride*, B.P., U.S.P., which forms colourless crystals soluble in water. It is very rarely given internally, 8–16 mg. ($\frac{1}{8}$–$\frac{1}{4}$ gr.). As a local anaesthetic it is used in varying strengths of solution, according to the depth and duration of anaesthesia required and the region to which it is applied. For example, to allay pain in the conjunctiva a 1 per cent. solution may suffice, whereas for complete anaesthesia of the eye 4 per cent. may be necessary. Stronger solutions may be applied to limited areas of the nose or larynx. Poisoning may occur from absorption from a mucous surface, especially from the nose or urethra.

The danger of habit-formation with cocaine must always be

kept in mind, though it is only likely to occur from repeated use. It is a habit which rapidly leads to mental and moral deterioration. *Habitués* usually take it as a snuff, for it is rapidly absorbed from the nasal mucous membrane, and so produces its action on the central nervous system. The chief symptoms arising from repeated indulgence in cocaine are loss of appetite, emaciation, sleeplessness, tremors, hallucinations, and finally more serious mental symptoms. The substitutes for cocaine do not seem to induce habit-formation.

Though the addition of adrenaline has materially reduced the dangers of cocaine injections, it has not entirely removed them. There remains still the danger, for example, of the combined solution accidentally entering a vein; and both adrenaline and cocaine are very much more toxic by intravenous than by hypodermic injection. Attempts have, therefore, been made to discover substances which would possess the local anaesthetic action of cocaine with a diminished general toxicity. Also, the dangers of habit-formation with cocaine and the widespread abuse of this drug have prompted the search for substitutes which would have no tendency to induce habit. Though much progress has been made in this direction, a local anaesthetic ideal for all purposes has not yet been discovered. Cocaine is still one of the best for producing surface anaesthesia, partly because it penetrates the mucous surface better than most anaesthetics, but less toxic substitutes have displaced it for other types of anaesthesia.

COCAINE SUBSTITUTES

Of the newer substitutes for cocaine the following may be mentioned.

Procaine Hydrochloride, B.P., U.S.P., is one of the most widely used and satisfactory substitutes for cocaine. It is much less toxic than cocaine and does not seem to induce habit-formation. It has the disadvantage, for many purposes, compared with cocaine, that it does not cause local constriction of the vessels, nor does it act so well as a surface anaesthetic because it less readily penetrates the mucous membrane. It is generally used as a solution combined with adrenaline for reasons already explained (p. 137). So used, it has largely replaced cocaine for all forms of injection anaesthesia. The alkaloidal base procaine is more actively anaesthetic than the hydrochloride but is too insoluble for use.

Lignocaine Hydrochloride, B.P., (Xylocaine, Lidocaine), was synthesized by Lofgren in Sweden in 1943, since when it has become extensively used. It is believed by many anaesthetists to be the most generally satisfactory local anaesthetic at present available. It is more stable than procaine in solution. The onset of anaesthesia is more rapid (in about $1-1\frac{1}{2}$ minutes) and the effect more lasting, than with procaine. Both substances have approximately the same toxicity. Lignocaine in actual use has a very low incidence of undesirable effects. It is used in solutions of 0·5–2 per cent. with or without adrenaline for infiltration and nerve blocks and in 2–4 per cent. solutions for surface anaesthesia. It does not irritate the cornea.

Amethocaine Hydrochloride, B.P., U.S.P., closely resembles procaine chemically and pharmacologically. It penetrates mucous membranes better and so can be used as a surface anaesthetic for the eye, nose, or throat. It is also used as a spinal anaesthetic.

Cinchocaine Hydrochloride, B.P., *Dibucaine Hydrochloride*, U.S.P., is more toxic than cocaine but, for most purposes, proportionately more active as a local anaesthetic and so can be used in weaker concentrations. Its action is also more prolonged. It is used to induce surface, infiltration, or spinal anaesthesia.

Butacaine Sulphate, B.P., is more toxic than cocaine by hypodermic injection and is not used for injection anaesthesia. It is used especially as a surface anaesthetic for the eye, acting more rapidly than cocaine, and, as weaker concentrations are effective, it is less toxic when so used.

Piperocaine Hydrochloride, U.S.P., is used for infiltration and spinal anaesthesia. Its toxicity is low.

Benzocaine, B.P., and *Butyl Aminobenzoate*, B.P., are both almost insoluble in water and are used chiefly as dusting powders, suitably diluted, to relieve the pain of burns, ulcers, fissures, &c. Benzocaine may also be used in the form of an ointment or suppository. They differ from the previous soluble compounds in producing less complete but more lasting local anaesthesia and with less risk of toxic effects.

Yet another type of local anaesthetic is *Ethyl Chloride* (p. 100).

Before the introduction of cocaine several other substances were used as surface local anaesthetics. For example, opium, belladonna, aconite, hydrocyanic acid, and menthol were all applied locally to the skin for the relief of pain. They are not very effective, and are now rarely used for this purpose.

XII

DRUGS ACTING AT EFFERENT
NERVE-ENDINGS

CHOLINERGIC NERVES

THE nerves which supply the voluntary muscles run uninter-
ruptedly from the central nervous system to the muscles, so
that, outside the central nervous system, the nerve supply of
the voluntary muscles is anatomically simple. The nerve supply
of involuntary muscles is, outside the central nervous system,
more complicated. In the first place the nerves emerging from
the central nervous system have their paths to the involuntary
muscles interrupted by ganglia and, secondly, each muscle
almost invariably receives a double nerve supply. When involuntary muscles throughout the body are compared it is
found that each of the two nerves supplying an organ conforms
to one or other of two anatomically distinct patterns. For this
and other reasons the nerves supplying involuntary muscle
have been classified into two divisions, to which the names
sympathetic and parasympathetic have been applied. The term
'autonomic nervous system' includes both these divisions,
which supply not only involuntary muscles but also most
secreting glands.

SYMPATHETIC AND PARASYMPATHETIC NERVES

The sympathetic nerves arise from the dorso-lumbar part
of the spinal cord; the parasympathetic from the mid-brain,
medulla oblongata, and sacral part of the spinal cord. The
peripheral ganglia of the parasympathetic nerves are usually
close to the organs they supply, those of the sympathetic nerves
remote from the organ, i.e. nearer to the central nervous
system. The parasympathetic nerves tend to find a place in the
larger nerve trunks which, being more noticeable, have received

special names, such as the oculomotor and vagus nerves. The sympathetic nerves, on the other hand, usually run in more numerous but small trunks.

Stimulation of the sympathetic nerve to an organ has usually an effect different from that of stimulation of its parasympathetic nerve, e.g. stimulation of the cardiac sympathetic nerve causes acceleration and augmentation of the heart, whereas stimulation of the vagus causes slowing and depression. In the case of the heart, therefore, the nerves are physiological antagonists, and so they are usually. One of the chief difficulties in regard to the autonomic nervous system is, however, that though the sympathetic and the parasympathetic nerves to a particular organ usually have antagonistic actions, it is not always the sympathetic nerve which is the motor one and the parasympathetic the inhibitor (as in the heart), for, in the case of the bronchi for example, the vagus is the motor and the sympathetic nerve the inhibitor nerve. Hence a drug like adrenaline has a motor effect on some organs and an inhibitor effect on others, depending on what happens to be the effect of sympathetic stimulation on the particular organ.

Though this division of the autonomic nervous system into sympathetic and parasympathetic nerves has a real basis and is still a classification convenient for certain purposes, work on the humoral transmission of nerve impulses has led to a parallel and perhaps more significant classification based upon the particular chemical transmitter which is discharged at the nerve-ends in muscles and ganglia.

ADRENERGIC AND CHOLINERGIC NERVES

When a postganglionic fibre of a sympathetic nerve is stimulated, or when any effective stimulus passes through it, noradrenaline with a small proportion of adrenaline is liberated at the nerve-ending, and the effect produced is due to the action of these on the muscle fibre.

The functional arrangement is such that the effects of stimulating postganglionic parasympathetic nerves are usually localized whereas the effects of stimulating postganglionic sympathetic nerves are more diffuse. This feature is reinforced by the discharge from the medulla of the adrenal gland of a mixture of adrenaline and its congener noradrenaline, which passes via the blood stream to all organs and tissues and re-inforces the general effects of sympathetic nervous activity, especially during emergency.

It had long been known that the effects produced by adrena-line and the effects produced by peripheral sympathetic stimu-lation were similar, and this is now explained by the fact that the latter effects are also due to adrenaline and noradrenaline. The actions of adrenaline were formerly described as a 'stimu-lation of sympathetic nerve-ends'. This is not strictly correct because adrenaline produces its effects by combining with some chemical receptor not in the nerve-endings but in the muscle, and will in fact act when the nerves to the muscles have de-generated.

When a postganglionic fibre of a parasympathetic nerve is stimulated, acetylcholine is liberated at the nerve-ends and the effect produced is due to the action of the acetylcholine, so liberated, upon the muscle. Acetylcholine acts as a chemical transmitter of peripheral parasympathetic nerve impulses in the same way as noradrenaline does for peripheral sympathetic nerve impulses. Whereas the latter is the sole known function of noradrenaline as a transmitter, acetylcholine has a winer sphere of action because it also acts as a chemical transmitter of impulses passing from all preganglionic fibres of the auto-nomic system (sympathetic and parasympathetic) to the nerve ganglia and also of those passing from the somatic nerves to the voluntary muscles. Nerves which act by liberation of noradrenaline and adrenaline are called adrenergic nerves, those which act by liberation of acetylcholine, cholinergic nerves.

Though acetylcholine stimulates voluntary and involuntary muscle as well as autonomic ganglia, it may be supposed that the receptors in those different tissues with which it combines are not identical or equally accessible. In that event it might happen that other drugs might combine with one or more of these receptors and so reproduce part or whole of the effects of acetylcholine. Actually this is the case, whatever may be the explanation. Muscarine, an alkaloid obtained from a poisonous mushroom (*Amanita muscaria*), and chemically related to acetylcholine, has a more restricted sphere of action than acetylcholine as it stimulates only the tissues supplied by the postganglionic fibres of the parasympathetic nerves. Drugs which have a stimulating action at this site can be conveniently described as having a 'muscarine action'.

Nicotine, an alkaloid occurring in tobacco, selects the other sites influenced by acetylcholine, for it stimulates voluntary muscle and autonomic ganglia. Drugs which reproduce this group of actions are said to have a 'nicotine action'. The actions of acetylcholine, therefore, can be described as a combination of muscarine and nicotine actions. Muscarine actions are antagonized by atropine, nicotine effects by curare and by large doses of nicotine itself.

Similarly, drugs other than adrenaline, for the most part near relatives of adrenaline, are known which stimulate the same structures as adrenaline and are sometimes called 'sympathomimetic', as their effects resemble those produced by stimulation of the sympathetic nerves. Some of these effects, especially motor effects, are antagonized by ergotoxine, &c.

It is now believed that, normally in the body, acetylcholine acts as a chemical transmitter of nerve impulses in three regions: (1) the terminations of all motor nerves to voluntary muscles (2) the terminations of all preganglionic nerve fibres; (3) the terminations of postganglionic fibres of parasympathetic nerves. In addition it is thought that acetylcholine plays some part in the activity of the central nervous system. When suitably applied to isolated organs or when injected into a vein in an intact animal, acetylcholine can reproduce the effects of stimulation of all three groups of nerve fibres mentioned above. Certain drugs which produce one or more of the three group-actions may now be considered with special reference to those which are used therapeutically.

A. SKELETAL MUSCLE (MOTOR NERVES)

I. *STIMULANTS*

Nicotine stimulates and, in larger doses, paralyses voluntary muscles, this being part of the complex of effects designated 'nicotine action'. Impulses passing down the motor nerve bring about release of acetylcholine at the region of the motor end plate or neuromuscular junction. The effect of this labile substance, which diffuses rapidly across the interfacial gap between nerve-end and muscle cell and which bears a heavily charged quaternary ammonium ion, is to alter the electrical charge on the surface of the muscle cell (depolarization). Processes which are initiated by this change result in contraction of the muscle fibre. The acetylcholine is quickly destroyed by the enzyme cholinesterase of which there are in man two forms, a specific cellular enzyme and a more generally distributed pseudo-cholinesterase. The muscle cell membrane returns to normal, preparatory to the whole process being repeated. Fusion of repetitive short-lasting contractions produces the smooth 'tetanus' of normal muscle activity. Associated with the release of acetylcholine there is a movement of potassium ions, the significance of which is obscure.

It follows that acetylcholine itself (p. 157) will cause a contraction of muscle, but in practice this will only occur if it is administered by 'close arterial injection', as by any other route the cholinesterase will destroy it before it is effective. If larger amounts are injected this stimulation may be followed by depression and the muscle becomes temporarily inexcitable to a nerve impulse. This effect is due to excessive depolarization, the transference of nerve impulses involving re-polarization alternately with depolarization. Acetylcholine can thus be said (pharmacologically) to stimulate motor nerve-ends to voluntary muscle in small doses and to paralyse them in larger ones. Under normal conditions of functioning only the former action comes into play. Also the choline esters carbachol and methacholine (p. 158) have similar effects.

ANTICHOLINESTERASES

A similar result may be brought about by inhibiting the destructive effect of cholinesterase enzyme by the action of one or other of the anticholinesterase drugs. These are the following:

Physostigmine Salicylate, B.P., U.S.P. (Eserine Salicylate), is described in detail on p. 158. Any substance which inhibits true cholinesterase will enhance all the actions of acetylcholine, both muscarine and nicotine types. The former type of activity is more augmented by physostigmine than is the latter. Its clinical use is, therefore, to produce muscarine-like effects and accordingly it is described with the stimulants of postganglionic parasympathetic activity. Nevertheless it prolongs or intensifies the effect of the normal transmission of nerve impulses to voluntary muscle in adequate amounts and in gross excess produces weakness of the muscle or even paralysis.

Myasthenia gravis is a disease characterized by a relative failure to produce or to release adequate amounts of acetylcholine at neuromuscular junctions. The main feature is that of increasing fatigue and muscular weakness on exercise, which may be so severe as to endanger life. Physostigmine has a dramatic effect in temporarily relieving the paresis by protection of the released acetylcholine from its specific enzyme. The undesired muscarine actions of physostigmine are such that efforts were made to improve upon it.

Neostigmine may be administered orally as *Neostigmine Bromide*, B.P., U.S.P., 15–30 mg., or by injection as *Neostigmine Methylsulphate*, B.P., 0·5–2 mg., U.S.P., 0·25–1 mg. Structurally it is related to physostigmine but is of synthetic origin. It is a quaternary ammonium compound, and like all such, is poorly absorbed when given by mouth or applied locally to membranes. It is chiefly notable for the speedy, reversible inhibition of cholinesterase which it produces and the dominance of the nicotinic cholinergic response which ensues. Effects on the central nervous system are seen if poisoning with it occurs, and muscarinic actions such as slowing of the pulse rate, constriction of the pupil, and increase in intestinal peristalsis, &c., are readily obtainable, but it is the drug of choice in the diagnosis and treatment of myasthenia. This is in part due to the fact that neostigmine, as a carbamic acid ester, exerts some direct stimulant action on muscle fibres, of a cholinergic type. Abuse by overdosage produces muscular weakness, as with physostigmine.

Another group of anticholinesterases exists which differ from physostigmine and neostigmine in their structure (they contain phosphorus), in the fact that they preferentially inhibit non-specific or pseudo-cholinesterase and that the inhibition is irreversible. Clinically their chief effects are muscarine-like and accordingly they are described with physostigmine (p. 160) but they are capable of exerting nicotinic actions. They are not used therapeutically for this purpose.

Potassium chloride (p. 31) causes a contraction of voluntary muscle when applied to suitable preparations but little use can be made of this property. The shift of potassium ions is coincidental with muscle contraction rather than of primary importance to neuromuscular conduction but muscular weakness is a feature of potassium loss and is relieved by potassium chloride given orally.

Ephedrine (p. 172) and certain other sympathomimetic amines have a beneficial effect in myasthenia by facilitating the response of muscle fibres to acetylcholine.

II. *DEPRESSANTS*

CURARIFORM DRUGS

About the middle of the eighteenth century, attention began to be directed to the use of an arrow poison by the South American Indians, in the regions of the Amazon, Dutch Guiana, and elsewhere. Travellers had witnessed the rapid death of animals struck by arrows having their tips smeared with a poison, now called curare. Actually Sir Walter Raleigh had known of the poison and brought some to Europe, but little came of it.

There are some interesting points about the use of this substance as an arrow poison. It rapidly produces paralysis of voluntary muscles, including the respiratory muscles. The speed of effect would depend on the amount absorbed and the size and species of animal, but it was an effective type of poison for preventing the animal's escape. It has little action when swallowed and therefore the flesh of an animal killed by it could be eaten with impunity.

The classical experiments of Claude Bernard showed that, when a muscle was exposed to the action of curare, stimulation of the nerve failed to produce contraction of the muscle, though the muscle was still quite excitable when stimulated directly. His experiments were important not only from his correct conclusion that curare must paralyse conduction of the nerve-ends but also as they were one of the first successful types of experiment designed to elucidate the precise site of action of a drug.

Curare was tried medicinally in diseases like epilepsy, tetanus, &c., in which, by its type of action, it might be expected to suppress excessive muscular contractions, but, partly owing to the variability in potency of different specimens of curare, it proved an unreliable remedy and had to await the isolation of an active principle for it to attain an established therapeutic use. Curares from different districts of South America were named according to the type of container—earthenware pots, gourds, or tubes—and from tube-curare a pure alkaloid, tubocurarine, was isolated which has now supplanted crude preparations. This, in the form of *Tubocurarine Chloride*, B.P., U.S.P., is widely used to produce relaxation of skeletal muscle during anaesthesia (p. 103), being injected intravenously in doses of 15 mg. The development of the full effect takes 5–10 minutes and persists for another hour. Since the mode of action is to raise the threshold of the muscle fibre membrane to depolarization by acetylcholine it follows that curare is antagonized by anticholinesterases which increase the amount of available acetylcholine. In practice 3 mg. of Neostigmine Methylsulphate is injected as an antidote to terminate the effects of curare after the operative procedure has finished. Curare does not readily distinguish between one skeletal muscle and another but there is some slight 'sparing' of the diaphragm. Nevertheless respiratory paralysis is very readily produced and the therapeutic index of the drug is far too low to permit of its use unless full control of respiration has been instituted. With this precaution toxicity is very low although a degree of cerebral stimulation occurs, and too rapid injection may cause a fall in blood pressure and constriction of the bronchi from release of tissue histamine. Curare does not antagonize the muscarinic actions of acetylcholine. In amounts some ten times greater than those needed to cause muscular paralysis it blocks conduction from pre- to postganglionic neurones in the autonomic ganglia. This effect may give rise to loss of vascular tone and oozing of blood from cut surfaces.

Gallamine Triethiodide, B.P., dose: determined in accordance with the patient's needs (usually about 80 mg.), is a synthetic substance of simpler structure than curare, but like it a quaternary ammonium derivative. It produces the same effects and acts in the same way but presents certain differences in detail. This substance is less potent, the paralysis is of quicker onset (3 minutes) and its duration, due to rapid excretion, is much less. It has a relatively greater ganglion blocking effect and thus causes a rapid pulse by blocking the vagus nerve. Like curare it is synergistic with ether and with chlorpromazine. It is preferable for short operations where tachycardia is not of importance.

Some 80 per cent. of patients are given these agents to facilitate endotracheal intubation and in about half the paralysis is continued to aid surgery. Gallamine is antagonized by neostigmine.

PERSISTENT DEPOLARIZING AGENTS

It has already been explained that excess of acetylcholine at the neuromuscular junction results in persistent depolarization of the membrane which interrupts what is essentially an alternating process. It is scarcely surprising therefore that compounds exist which resemble acetylcholine in structure closely enough to bring about this depolarizing effect but which are not destroyed by cholinesterase. They therefore paralyse muscle. The first of these to be tried was a symmetrical synthetic structure in which a 10-carbon methylene chain separates identical quaternary ammonium groups—*Decamethonium Iodide*, B.P. This type of structure will be seen again (p. 153), but C10, as the compound is sometimes called, fell into disuse because of the difficulty in controlling its effects.

Suxamethonium Chloride, B.P., *Succinylcholine Chloride*, U.S.P., is given as a sterile intravenous *Injection of Suxamethonium Chloride*, B.P., in doses of 10–40 mg. or more. It produces an immediate paralysis which has the merit of brevity (2–4 minutes). This feature is due to the fact that the compound is only slowly resistant to the effects of cholinesterase. In some patients enzyme is deficient and the paralysis becomes a long one. There is no antidote, anticholinesterases such as neostigmine augmenting the paralysis (contrast with curare and gallamine). The means of assisting respiration must be available before it may be used. Like all depolarizing agents it causes a brief interlude of fasciculation or stimulation of muscle before paralysis sets in. It is used to control electroconvulsion therapy and to facilitate intubation for anaesthesia. Patients may complain of stiffness after its use.

The general anaesthetic ether has a depressant effect on neuromuscular conduction and so has chlorpromazine which is sometimes used during anaesthesia. The dosage of 'relaxants' may have to be adjusted accordingly.

Quinine (p. 296) has some curare-like action and also increases the refractory period of voluntary muscle, so that the effect of a tetanus is diminished. For these actions quinine is beneficial in a rare disease, myotonia congenita, in which voluntary movements are impeded by undue prolongation of muscular contraction.

B. AUTONOMIC GANGLIA (PREGANGLIONIC NERVES)

I. *STIMULANTS*

Nicotine stimulates both sympathetic and parasympathetic nerve ganglia. As these nerves have usually opposite actions on involuntary muscle, the resultant effects are complex and are rendered more complicated by the fact that nicotine later paralyses both these ganglia. By this latter effect it prevents the stimulant action of acetylcholine on ganglia. The actions of nicotine are too complex and vary too much with small changes in dosage for this alkaloid to be used therapeutically. Lobeline, an alkaloid obtained from lobelia, has actions very similar to those of nicotine. It has been used as a respiratory stimulant, acting through the carotid sinus (p. 81).

All choline esters have nicotine as well as muscarine actions, particularly acetylcholine (p. 157); and anticholinesterases produce a similar effect by allowing an accumulation of acetylcholine. Their muscarine actions if not prevented mask their actions on the ganglia. Potassium salts and adrenaline exert facilitating actions on the ganglia similar to those on the neuromuscular functions.

NICOTINE

Though nicotine has practically no place in therapeutics, tobacco which owes its effects mainly to nicotine, is of great importance from its world-wide use and from the effects it may produce. These may now be mentioned.

Tobacco

From the time of Columbus, who first learnt of the use of tobacco from the natives of San Salvador, the indulgence in leaf tobacco (smoked, chewed, or snuffed) has spread over the world, and has been at times extolled as a panacea for diseases and at times execrated as a highly noxious vice. A gigantic 'experiment' has been made on millions of people for over four centuries, and the modest conclusion can be drawn that the results on human health and longevity have, at any rate so far, not been calamitous. This is not to say that the habit of smoking, which is by far the commonest form of indulgence, can be entirely exonerated of harmful effects.

A beginner's introduction to the delights of smoking often

takes the form of nausea, vomiting, slow pulse, cold sweats, and faintness, mainly due to stimulation of the vagus and vomiting centres. With practice these centres become appeased, but similar symptoms may affect even the habitual smoker as a result of over-indulgence.

The pleasures of smoking are complicated, partly due to the ritual associated with it and often to the fact that it is a social habit (any common practice tending to bring people *en rapport* with one another), but there can be little doubt that the dominant factor is the absorption of nicotine and its pharmacological effects on the individual. As far as effects are concerned which suggest actions on the central nervous system, people vary greatly in what they think they get out of smoking. Some people find it soothing, possibly most likely to occur if nicotine is more leisurely absorbed, as in pipe-smoking; others find it stimulating, especially cigarette-smokers, who probably get a quicker rise of nicotine in the blood. A pharmacological explanation of these differences in terms of the known actions of nicotine on the central nervous system is somewhat elusive. Here only a brief summary can be given of the accredited effects of tobacco, which naturally vary with the amount used and the method, and with the degree of tolerance established.

Tobacco produces a transient rise of blood pressure, increased rate of the heart and constriction of some peripheral vessels, with a fall in skin temperature. It may produce a temporary reduction in urinary secretion due to stimulation of the supraoptic nucleus with resulting liberation of the antidiuretic hormone of the posterior pituitary lobe. Possibly this hormone may also produce some coronary constriction. In some people smoking may produce palpitation or anginal pain. People with occlusive vascular disease especially thromboangiitis obliterans and possibly those with coronary disease should avoid smoking.

The irritant effect of tobacco smoke (due to other constituents as well as nicotine) may irritate the pharynx and larynx and aggravate coughing. It is claimed that smoking reduces vital capacity and chest expansion, which may justify the general belief that smoking is 'bad for the wind' and not good for athletes. Smoking, especially of strong tobacco in pipes, may produce amblyopia, usually in middle-aged men, with malnutrition as a predisposing cause. Among other effects which may result from excessive smoking are palpitations, tremor, and nervousness.

In recent years a more important question has arisen over a possible connexion between increased consumption of tobacco and cancer of the lung which has shown such a remarkable coincident increase in prevalence and mortality. An inescapable relation has been shown between smoking, especially heavy and long-continued smoking of cigarettes, and the incidence of lung cancer. This relation is at present only statistical since no incriminating carcinogenic agent has yet been found in tobacco smoke. The evidence suggests that there are additionally other factors responsible, but a partial conclusion seems to be warranted—one who does not smoke cigarettes will be much less likely to suffer in later years from cancer of the lung.

II. DEPRESSANTS

The paralysing action of decamethonium has already been mentioned (p. 150). Reduction of the number of methylene groups from 10 in decamethonium to 6 in hexamethonium or 5 in pentolinium produces compounds that act mainly as ganglion blocking agents.

GANGLION BLOCKING DRUGS

Hexamethonium Tartrate, B.P., blocks conduction through both sympathetic and parasympathetic ganglia. Its therapeutic value is due to the former action. By interruption of sympathetic vasomotor tone, it lowers blood pressure and increases blood flow especially in the lower limbs. Since reflex response to alteration in posture is diminished, the fall of pressure is greater when the patient is in the upright position, when faintness, relieved by lying down, may occur. Hexamethonium is feebly and somewhat erratically absorbed from the alimentary canal and parenteral injection gives the more reliable results. Even so, different patients vary in their response to the same dose and the dosage necessary to produce the desired degree of lowering of blood pressure must be carefully estimated for each patient. The onset of ganglion block is rapid and usually persists for 3–8 hours. By reducing hypertension, hexamethonium can relieve or abolish the severe headaches, breathlessness, and palpitation which accompany the condition. It may prevent loss of sight by reversing retinitis and papilloedema, and in many cases probably prolongs life.

Unfortunately the block is not confined to the sympathetic ganglia and simultaneous block of the parasympathetic ganglia may have undesired but unavoidable effects, which in some cases may make continuation of treatment difficult. These include dryness of the mouth and throat, making speech and swallowing difficult, blurred vision due to dilatation of the pupil and paralysis of accommodation, stasis of the bowel and retention of urine.

Pentolinium Tartrate is so similar to hexamethonium both in its therapeutic effects and side-effects that no separate description of it is necessary. It is more active than hexamethonium so that smaller doses are required. It has been specially recommended for oral administration.

Many other drugs have been tried in recent years to lower blood pressure in hypertension though probably none is so reliable in severe hypertension with retinal changes as the methonium compounds. Two of the most frequently used drugs may be taken here because, though they do not act by paralysing ganglia, they are used as adjuvants to, or sometimes substitutes for, the methonium compounds.

RAUWOLFIA. Extracts of *Rauwolfia serpentina*, and, more recently, one of its alkaloids *Reserpine* (used also as a sedative, p. 110) are used in the treatment of hypertension. As Rauwolfia does not interfere with transmission at autonomic ganglia, and is neither adrenolytic nor sympatholytic, it has been suggested that it acts on the hypothalamus. Full benefit from its action is not observed until it has been given for 2 or 3 weeks. In mild cases of hypertension it may prove satisfactory alone, but usually it is given along with hexamethonium or now perhaps more frequently with pentolinium whereby a sufficient and steadier depressor effect can be obtained with smaller doses of the latter drugs. Side-effects with Rauwolfia include nasal congestion, drowsiness, and bradycardia, but these symptoms often abate with continued use.

VERATRUM ALKALOIDS can produce a significant lowering of pressure in a considerable proportion of hypertensive patients. Veratrum has long had a place in the treatment of acute blood pressure rises in eclampsia. Veratrum and its alkaloids act by inducing reflex vasodilatation, the afferent fibres arising in the coronary vascular bed.

C. PARASYMPATHETIC NERVE-ENDINGS (POSTGANGLIONIC NERVES)

I. STIMULANTS

The part played by acetylcholine in the transmission of nervous impulses has already been explained. The 'nicotine actions' (stimulation of voluntary muscle and ganglia) are less pronounced than the 'muscarine actions' (stimulation of tissues supplied by postganglionic parasympathatic fibres), and consequently the actions of acetylcholine closely resemble those of muscarine. Several other alkaloids (e.g. pilocarpine, arecoline) produce this muscarine type of action, which has usually been described as a stimulation of parasympathetic nerve-ends, though, as has been previously explained, they actually stimulate the peripheral tissue itself, rather than the nerve-endings.

The effects produced by drugs of this group ('muscarine actions') closely resemble those produced by stimulation of all the parasympathetic nerves. They have a few additional actions, especially stimulation of the sweat glands, the nerves to which, though belonging anatomically to the sympathetic, resemble the parasympathetic in liberating acetylcholine in response to stimulation. The tissues innervated by the autonomic nervous system consist mainly of involuntary muscle and glands, and the actions of this group of drugs on a particular organ can be predicted provided one knows the effect on it of stimulation of its parasympathetic nerve. This group of actions can be more usefully described under pilocarpine than under muscarine, as the latter alkaloid is not used in practical therapeutics.

Pilocarpine, an alkaloid obtained from *Pilocarpus microphyllus* produces effects similar to simultaneous stimulation of all the parasympathetic nerves. Only the more important of these effects need be mentioned.

In regard to *involuntary muscle*, pilocarpine causes contraction of the sphincter pupillae and therefore makes the pupil smaller; it also causes contraction of the ciliary muscle, thereby fixing accommodation at the focus for short distance; intraocular tension is lowered after a preliminary rise. These effects on the eye are produced not only when pilocarpine circulates in the blood but also when it is applied in solution to the conjunctiva. Pilocarpine slows the heart, constricts the bronchi, and augments the movements of the stomach and intestine. The bladder muscle is also stimulated.

In regard to *glands*, pilocarpine stimulates the secretion of the salivary, buccal, bronchial, lachrymal, and enteric glands. It also stimulates the sweat glands. It does not increase the secretion of urine or milk.

Once pilocarpine enters the circulation, it acts on all these organs, but in the smallest effective doses it acts more on glands than on smooth muscle. With the latter doses, therefore, the chief noticeable symptoms are increased salivation, sweating, and bronchial secretion. Larger doses may slow the heart and augment the movements of the stomach and intestine, and may produce vomiting and diarrhoea. Poisonous doses embarrass the respiration (from constriction of the bronchi and blocking of their lumen by secretion) as well as the circulation (from cardiac slowing). In many animals convulsions precede death.

From what has already been said, it will be intelligible that pilocarpine is used mainly for stimulating gland secretions. It must be used with care, but with smallest doses the action on glands can be obtained without any serious cardiac slowing or bronchial constriction. It is used chiefly for increasing sweat secretion in serious diseases of the kidney, for it is one of the most powerful of known diaphoretics; less frequently it is used as an expectorant, for which effect there are numerous and safer substitutes. Though, in prescribing it, one may desire only its diaphoretic action, it is not easy to escape its action on the bronchial and other glands, and this is often a disadvantage as compared with other methods of producing diaphoresis.

The official salt of pilocarpine is *Pilocarpine Nitrate*, B.P., 3–12 mg. ($\frac{1}{20}$–$\frac{1}{5}$ gr.), U.S.P., 5–20 mg.

Arecoline, an alkaloid obtained from Betel Nut, has actions similar to pilocarpine, but is not used in regular medicine.

CHOLINE ESTERS

Choline has the formula $(CH_3)_3 \equiv N(OH)CH_2 \cdot CH_2OH$.

Various esters of choline are physiologically much more active than choline itself.

ACETYLCHOLINE

Acetylcholine, in which the H of the terminal hydroxyl group is replaced by $COCH_3$, is about 1,000 times more active than choline. Acetylcholine exerts both muscarine and nicotine actions (p. 144), the former being more prominent. Its actions, therefore, closely resemble those of pilocarpine, already described (p. 156). It is rapidly hydrolysed in the body into choline and acetic acid by esterases in the blood and tissues and its activity proportionally reduced. Its effects are too transient for it to have much place in therapeutics, but some other choline esters which are more stable have proved of greater medicinal value.

Carbachol, B.P., U.S.P., (Carbamylcholine Chloride), in which the H of the terminal hydroxyl group of choline is replaced by $CONH_2$, has a more prolonged action than acetylcholine and is active when given orally or by parenteral injection. It has been used to stimulate the involuntary muscle in paralytic conditions of the bladder and intestine and by application in solution to the conjunctiva, to constrict the pupil and to lower intraocular tension in glaucoma. It must be given with care. It may cause cardiac slowing, fall of blood pressure, flushing, sweating, nausea, constriction of bronchi—symptoms that one would expect from its type of action. Doses, B.P., oral 1–4 mg., subcutaneous 0·25–0·5 mg.; U.S.P., topically, $\frac{3}{4}$–1$\frac{1}{2}$ per cent. solution or ointment.

Methacholine Chloride, B.P., U.S.P., (acetyl-β-methylcholine Chloride), has a profound effect in slowing the rate of and conduction in the heart, dilating peripheral vessels, and thus lowering blood pressure. Dose, B.P., oral, 0·1–0·2 G., subcutaneous, 10–25 mg.; U.S.P., subcutaneous, 20 mg. It is destroyed rapidly by cell cholinesterase but not by plasma enzyme. The chief clinical application of these actions is in the treatment of severe paroxysmal tachycardia which will not yield to other therapy. They have proved disappointing in other fields but may be used to counter intestinal atony or acute retention of urine where there is no mechanical blockage.

Bethanechol Chloride, U.S.P., (Carbamylmethylcholine Chloride), 10 mg. three times a day by mouth, 2·5 mg. by injection, has similar actions to methacholine but is not a ganglionic stimulant and is resistant to the action of cholinesterase.

ANTICHOLINESTERASES

Physostigmine (Eserine) is an alkaloid obtained from the seeds of *Physostigma venenosum* (calabar bean), a tall climbing plant growing round the Gulf of Guinea. The calabar bean was used by the tribes of Tropical West Africa as an 'ordeal' poison. It was introduced into modern medicine in 1863 for constricting the pupil.

Physostigmine produces effects which closely resemble those of pilocarpine previously described (p. 156), but these effects are produced in a different way. It combines with cholinesterase and inhibits reversibly the action of this enzyme, which then can no longer hydrolyse acetylcholine. Consequently the actions of acetylcholine are prolonged and enhanced by physostigmine. This intensifying effect can be shown on an isolated tissue, such as the muscle of the leech, or *in vivo* by the fact that a given dose of acetylcholine causes a greater effect after physostigmine than before. When given by itself physostigmine causes positive effects, presumably because, by preventing hydrolysis of the acetylcholine normally liberated from the nerve-ends, it acts virtually as if added acetylcholine were being administered. It naturally therefore has both the muscarine and nicotine actions of acetylcholine (p. 144), but, as with the latter compound, the muscarine actions are more pronounced.

Toxic doses of physostigmine produce, as one would expect from its action, complicated effects arising from cardiac slowing, broncho-constriction, and violent contractions of the alimentary canal. In addition it paralyses the central nervous system, causing death mainly by respiratory failure.

Physostigmine is chiefly used for its action on the eye. Applied to the conjunctiva, it diffuses through and stimulates the 'ends' of the third nerve in (*a*) the sphincter pupillae and (*b*) the ciliary muscle. It therefore (*a*) contracts the pupil, and (*b*) produces spasm of accommodation, the contraction of the ciliary muscle fixing accommodation at the focus for short distance. But physostigmine is not used therapeutically for these effects so much as for its indirect effect in lowering intraocular pressure in diseases such as glaucoma, where the intraocular tension is dangerously high. This fall of pressure may last about 12 hours, and is generally ascribed to the opening up of the spaces of Fontana (by the contraction of the pupil) allowing freer escape of fluid.

Another important use of physostigmine is to stimulate the movements of the intestine. It is thus used, by hypodermic injection and especially in combination with pituitary (posterior lobe extract) to rouse the dormant contractions of the gut in post-operative intestinal atony.

The use of physostigmine in the treatment of muscular paralysis has already been referred to (p. 146). The official salt is *Physostigmine Salicylate*, B.P., 0·6–1·2 mg. ($\frac{1}{100}$–$\frac{1}{50}$ gr.), U.S.P., 2 mg., by mouth. For application to the eye, physostigmine is commonly used in a solution of 0·1–1·0 per cent., or as *Lamellae of Physostigmine*, B.P., containing 0·065 mg. in each.

Neostigmine, a compound having a structure similar to, but simpler than, that of physostigmine, resembles it also in pharmacological actions but is more stable. It is used in myasthenia gravis (p. 146) and in intestinal atony.

Isoflurophate, U.S.P., known in Britain by the approved name **Dyflos** (DFP), di*iso*propyl fluorophosphonate, is a colourless oily liquid with a characteristic odour. It is one of a group of organic alkyl phosphates which combine irreversibly with cholinesterases. DFP has a preferential affinity for serum or pseudocholinesterase which it readily inhibits. Only after all or most of the serum cholinesterase is inactivated does it inhibit cell cholinesterase and only then do symptoms and signs of poisoning ensue. The onset of effects is slow but persistent and the actions are the same as those of physostigmine and neostigmine. The only practical therapeutic application is by local instillation of a solution of 0·01–0·1 per cent. into the conjunctival sac to produce myosis and reduction in intraocular tension in glaucoma, a disease characterized by a great increase in the fluid pressure in the anterior chamber of the eye, with consequent headache and possible blindness. A number of other alkyl phosphates are in use as insecticides and weedkillers and on occasions poisoning of agricultural workers may occur. This is characterized by dizziness, loss of vision, nausea, vomiting, diarrhoea, low blood pressure, and muscular weakness. Treatment is carried out with large doses of atropine.

II. *DEPRESSANTS*

ATROPINE

Atropine is the chief alkaloid found in the leaves and root of *Hyoscyamus muticus*, a plant of the family Solanaceae. Many other species belonging to this natural order contain either atropine or some nearly related alkaloid.

The plant received its name herba belladonna so early as the sixth century from its use, by the 'fine ladies' of Venice, for the purpose of imparting lustre to the eyes by dilating the pupil which is one of its main actions. Though the plant was recognized as a poison, it did not come to be used in medicine till late in the eighteenth century, when it began to be employed in whooping-cough and for its mydriatic action. Later it came to be used as a local anodyne. The actions of belladonna are due mainly to the atropine in it.

Atropine is composed of a tropine and tropic acid radicle, tropine very nearly resembling the ecgonine radicle in cocaine. Atropine is a mixture of dextro- and laevo-hyoscyamine. As is so often the case with alkaloids, the laevo compound is much more active than the dextro, so that the action of atropine is mainly that of the laevo half. As laevo-hyoscyamine is difficult to obtain pure and has not come into general use and has qualitatively much the same actions as atropine, we need consider here only the actions of the natural mixture of laevo- and dextro-hyoscyamine, viz. atropine.

Atropine renders those tissues which are supplied by post-ganglionic fibres of the parasympathetic nerves insensitive to the action of acetylcholine. It antagonizes the muscarine actions not only of acetylcholine but also of muscarine itself, pilocarpine, arecoline, and physostigmine. It has no such effect on the nicotine actions of acetylcholine. It has actions, therefore, opposite to those of pilocarpine, already described. Its actions have previously been described as due to a paralysis of parasympathetic nerve-ends, but it does not prevent the liberation of acetylcholine when a postganglionic nerve fibre is stimulated, and therefore cannot strictly be regarded as paralysing these nerve-ends; but the effects produced are substantially the same as if it did. It must prevent effective access of acetylcholine to the innervated cell.

By acting at the terminations of the third nerve in the sphincter pupillae, atropine dilates the pupil; the ciliary muscle, also supplied by this nerve, is likewise paralysed, leading to paralysis of accommodation, it being impossible to focus for near objects; intraocular tension is raised. These ocular effects occur either when atropine is applied locally to the conjunctiva or when it circulates in the blood. By acting at the terminations of the vagus, atropine produces the following effects. The heart is quickened, the bronchi are relaxed, and exaggerated movements of the alimentary canal are diminished. In regard to the heart, the vagal paralysis produced by atropine prevents inhibitory impulses from the vagus centre reaching the heart. The amount of acceleration produced will therefore depend upon the degree of inhibition present, which will vary according to the species and age of the animal.

Small doses of atropine may cause slowing of the pulse in man due to stimulation of the vagus centre, the dose being insufficient to paralyse the vagal terminations.

By acting at the terminations of the nerves of most secreting glands, e.g. salivary, bronchial, lachrymal, and sweat glands, atropine diminishes their secretion.

In addition to these peripheral actions, atropine also acts on the *central nervous system*, stimulating first the medullary centres and later the motor areas of the cortex. Toxic doses paralyse the central nervous system eventually, the respiratory centre failing first.

The symptoms of *poisoning* by belladonna or atropine are the result of (*a*) the peripheral and (*b*) the central actions described above. There is (*a*) dryness of the mouth and throat, with thirst and difficulty of swallowing and speaking; dryness of the skin sometimes with an erythematous rash; dilated pupils with indistinctness of vision due to paralysis of accommodation: and (*b*) restlessness and garrulousness and eventually even convulsive movements, due to stimulation of the motor areas of the brain. Later the central nervous system may be depressed, and the patient may become paralysed and, if the dose be fatal, die mainly from paralysis of the respiratory centre.

THERAPEUTIC USES OF ATROPINE. Atropine is used in ophthalmological work, e.g. to dilate the pupil for diagnostic purposes or to paralyse accommodation in inflammatory conditions of the iris. Larger quantities are needed to paralyse the ciliary muscle than suffice to paralyse the sphincter pupillae. Two drawbacks to atropine for many purposes are the slowness of development of its effect (15–30 minutes) and its prolonged action, for the pupil may not recover its normal size or reactivity for several days. The fact that atropine raises intra-ocular pressure must always be kept in mind, for this often precludes its use.

For its action at the vagal ends in the bronchi, atropine is sometimes used in spasmodic asthma (which is usually due to reflex spasm of the bronchi). The early use of it in whooping-cough, for which it is sometimes still employed, may find an explanation in the same action. Atropine can also be used to relieve colic or to prevent spasmodic contractions of the gut. It acts similarly on the urinary bladder, and is often useful in incontinence of urine when this is due to hyperexcitability of the bladder reflex.

For its action on glands, atropine is frequently used to diminish bronchial or sweat secretion before general anaesthesia, though pethidine (p. 120) may be preferred. Its action cannot be confined to one set of glands exclusively.

The official salt is *Atropine Sulphate*, B.P., 0·25–1 mg. ($\frac{1}{240}-\frac{1}{60}$ gr.), U.S.P., 0·5 mg. The B.P. contains an *Eye Ointment of Atropine* (1 per cent.) and *Lamellae of Atropine*. The latter are small gelatine discs for insertion in the conjunctival sac, each containing 0·065 mg. of Atropine Sulphate. They are not popular. Of *Belladonna* the Leaf is official in the B.P. and the U.S.P. For internal administration the *Tincture of Belladonna*, B.P., 0·6–2 ml. (10–30 min.), U.S.P., 0·6 ml., may be used in mixtures, or the *Dry Extract of Belladonna*, B.P., 15–60 mg. ($\frac{1}{4}$–1 gr.), in pills or tablets.

Many other plants, belonging like belladonna to the natural order Solanaceae, have been found also to contain atropine or alkaloids closely related to it. Of these plants the most important is *Hyoscyamus niger*, the leaves of which form the official *Hyoscyamus*, B.P., which contains two alkaloids, Hyoscyamine, resembling atropine in action, and Hyoscine.

Hyoscine, B.P., *Scopolamine*, U.S.P., resembles atropine in all its peripheral actions, and produces the effects on smooth muscle and on secretions which have been described under atropine. Hence it can be used, for example, as a mydriatic in the same way as atropine or homatropine. It differs from atropine, however, in its action on the central nervous system, which it depresses from the outset without the previous stimulation that is seen with atropine, and is in fact chiefly used as a cerebral sedative. It differs from most hypnotics in that it primarily depresses the motor rather than the sensory side of the brain, and it produces sleep with a marked diminution of motor excitability. It is used chiefly in controlling the excitement of insanity and delirium tremens or for relieving the rigidity and tremor of paralysis (p. 114). For such purposes *Hyoscine Hydrobromide* is usually given subcutaneously in doses of 0·3–0·6 mg. ($\frac{1}{200}$–$\frac{1}{100}$ gr.). Hyoscine is also used in combination with morphine to produce narcosis, amnesia, and analgesia (p. 103). It is useful, given orally as *Tablets of Hyoscine Hydrobromide*, B.P., 0·3–0·6 mg. ($\frac{1}{200}$–$\frac{1}{100}$ gr.), for the prevention of sea-sickness or air-sickness (p. 115). From the hyoscyamus leaves there are prepared *Tincture of Hyoscyamus*, B.P., 2–4 ml. (30–60 min.), and *Dry Extract of Hyoscyamus*, B.P., 16–60 mg. ($\frac{1}{4}$–1 gr.), used often to relieve colic or to allay irritability of the bladder.

Stramonium, B.P., the leaves of another solanaceous plant, has much the same actions and uses as hyoscyamus and has been largely used in the treatment of Parkinsonism (p. 113). Like hyoscine, it produces a dramatic improvement in the mental condition as well as relieving the rigidity of the muscles and the excessive salivation. The B.P. has a *Dry Extract of Stramonium*, 15–60 mg. ($\frac{1}{4}$–1 gr.), or, in Parkinsonism, larger doses of 60–500 mg. (1–8 gr.); *Liquid Extract of Stramonium*, 0·06–0·2 ml. (1–3 min.); and *Tincture of Stramonium*, 0·6–2 ml. (10–30 min.).

Homatropine, an artificial compound of tropine and mandelic acid, is used as a substitute for atropine in ophthalmic practice. When applied to the eye it dilates the pupil almost as quickly as atropine, but its action passes off much sooner, e.g. in about 24 hours. It is more convenient than atropine for examination of the eye, and has less tendency to increase intraocular pressure. It may be used in the form of a solution of *Homatropine Hydrobromide*, 1–4 per cent., or of *Lamellae of Homatropine*, B.P., 0·65 mg. ($\frac{1}{100}$ gr.), in each. *Homatropine*

Methylbromide, U.S.P., may be given in doses of 10 mg. orally.

The relative success of the substitution of mandelic acid for tropic acid which gave homatropine encouraged further attempts at synthesis. Of these *Eucatropine Hydrochloride*, which is the mandeloxy compound of tetramethylpiperidine-hydrochloride, is official in the U.S.P. It is weak, short-acting, and when applied to the eye in 2 per cent. solution may dilate the pupil without disturbing accommodation. *Methantheline Bromide*, U.S.P., and *Propantheline Bromide*, are xanthene-9-carboxylates, powerful spasmolytics with relatively feeble anti-muscarine properties. They may be given by mouth in doses of 15–50 mg. several times per day to relieve spasm and pain associated with peptic ulceration. They are apt to cause dizziness, dryness of the mouth, blurring of vision, and other atropine-like symptoms in some patients.

XIII

DRUGS ACTING AT EFFERENT
NERVE-ENDINGS

ADRENERGIC NERVES

1. *STIMULANTS*

ADRENALINE (EPINEPHRINE)

THE discovery by Oliver and Schafer in 1894 that intravenous injection of an extract of suprarenal gland caused a remarkable rise of blood pressure has been one of the most fertile starting-points for physiological research of the twentieth century. Subsequent researches have shown that this effect is due to the presence in suprarenal gland-extract of two active principles—adrenaline and noradrenaline. $\text{HO} \diagdown \diagup \text{HO} \diagup \cdot \text{CHOH} \cdot \text{CH}_2 \cdot \text{NHCH}_3$ The constitutional formula for adrenaline is:

and it has been synthesized artificially.

The adrenaline as it occurs in the suprarenal gland and elsewhere in the body is *l*-adrenaline, which is much more active than *d*-adrenaline.

It is now believed that, when the postganglionic fibres of a sympathetic nerve are stimulated a mixture, chiefly of noradrenaline but containing some adrenaline, is liberated at the nerve-ends and that the effect produced is due to the action of the mixture on the involuntary muscle or gland. The amines act as chemical transmitters of sympathetic nerve impulses in the same way as does acetylcholine for parasympathetic nerve impulses (p. 157). When applied to an isolated organ, adrenaline produces almost the same effect as does stimulation of the sympathetic nerve to that organ, the latter effect being due to adrenaline and noradrenaline. When adrenaline is injected into a vein it produces a great variety of effects such as would be produced by simultaneous stimulation of all the true sympathetic nerves. The various actions of adrenaline can be predicted, with almost complete exactness, provided one knows what are the organs which receive a sympathetic nerve supply and what are the effects of sympathetic stimulation upon them. The prediction would not, however, be quite exact because a few discrepancies are found to occur. For example, though the sweat glands are supplied by sympathetic nerves, adrenaline does not increase the secretion of sweat. These nerves, though belonging anatomically to the sympathetic system, are exceptional in liberating acetylcholine and not adrenaline. It would be a more accurate generalization to say that adrenaline stimulates all tissues which are supplied by adrenergic nerve fibres. Its actions were formerly described as a 'stimulation of sympathetic nerve-ends', but this simplification ignores a few exceptions such as the sweat glands and also fails to indicate that adrenaline, like acetylcholine, acts on the peripheral tissue rather than the nerve-endings.

For a substance to act as a chemical transmitter of nerve impulses it would seem imperative that it should be capable of rapid destruction in the body, otherwise the effect of a nerve impulse would often last longer than was necessary or advantageous.

Adrenaline and noradrenaline rapidly disappear when they enter the tissues. The precise mode of disposal is obscure but a part may be played by oxidative de-amination catalysed by the intracellular enzyme amine-oxidase. Recovery of some of the activity from red blood cells is possible after adding adrenaline or noradrenaline to blood, where it would appear to be stored. If large amounts of adrenaline are taken by mouth a proportion is excreted in the urine conjugated with sulphate but oral administration is ineffective for therapeutic purposes. Absorption is imperfect from the hypodermic tissues, partly owing to local vasoconstriction. When injected into the blood stream its action is brief.

The action of adrenaline on the heart and blood vessels may

be dealt with first, as being first both in historical and in therapeutic importance. The rise of blood pressure produced by adrenaline is steep and high, but lasts only for a few minutes. It is partly due to contraction of the arterioles, as can be shown by the fact that the rise of pressure is accompanied by a diminution of intestinal volume. Adrenaline contracts blood vessels when applied locally to them or when perfused through an organ removed from the nervous system, i.e. it is a peripheral action. The vasoconstrictor supply to the heart, lungs, and brain is feeble or absent, and, correspondingly, adrenaline produces little or no constriction of the vessels to these organs. Therapeutic amounts injected in man probably lower the total peripheral resistance of the body due to the dilating effect of such amounts on the vessels of the skeletal muscles.

The isolated perfused mammalian or batrachian heart is augmented and accelerated by adrenaline, just as by stimulation of the cardiac sympathetic nerve. In the intact animal, however, especially at the height of the rise of blood pressure, the heart may be slowed. This is due to reflex slowing of the heart produced by the rise of pressure, which may overcome the direct effect of adrenaline on the heart itself. In man therapeutic doses usually quicken the pulse whereas noradrenaline slows the heart rate.

On involuntary muscle elsewhere adrenaline also produces effects like sympathetic stimulation. Injected intravenously it dilates the pupil. It dilates the bronchi if they are not already completely dilated. The splanchnic nerve (the sympathetic nerve to the alimentary canal) sends inhibitory fibres to the stomach and intestine, with the exception of the pyloric and ileocolic sphincters and the muscularis mucosae, to which the fibres are motor; similarly, adrenaline inhibits the tone and movements of the alimentary canal generally, but increases the contractions of these sphincters and of the muscularis mucosae.

The action of adrenaline on the uterus differs in different species of animals. Thus the uterus of the rabbit contracts, while the uterus of the guinea-pig and rat relaxes, in both instances whether the uteri are pregnant or not. The uterus of the cat contracts only when pregnant and relaxes when not pregnant. In each case the same effect is produced by stimulation of the sympathetic (hypogastric) nerve in these animals. The intact pregnant human uterus contracts to single intravenous doses of adrenaline but continued infusion causes relaxation; noradrenaline always causes contraction.

On glands the action of adrenaline is not so important as is that of acetylcholine or pilocarpine, for, generally, glandular secretions are influenced less by sympathetic than by parasympathetic stimulation. Adrenaline causes hyperglycaemia and glycosuria, by promoting glycogenolysis in the liver.

THERAPEUTIC USES OF ADRENALINE. Adrenaline is widely used as a local haemostatic. For example, it can be applied to the nasal mucous membrane to stop bleeding from the nose. It stops bleeding by causing extreme constriction of both arteries and veins. Its use with local anaesthetics has already been referred to (p. 137).

It may be used to raise blood pressure and stimulate the heart in some kinds of circulatory failure (but not in that occurring in the early stages of chloroform anaesthesia, when it may add to the risk of ventricular fibrillation). Though in the normal animal adrenaline produces only a very transient rise of pressure, in some abnormal conditions of low pressure it may produce a lasting rise. It is valuable in urticaria, angioneurotic oedema, and serum rash, probably from its vasomotor actions. It is used in that variety of asthma which is due to spasmodic contraction of the bronchioles. It is to be remembered that adrenaline has little or no effect on the blood pressure when given by mouth. This is due chiefly to its rapid destruction in the alimentary canal.

For parenteral injection, the B.P. has *Injection of Adrenaline*, a sterile, 1 in 1,000, solution of Adrenaline Acid Tartrate, stabilized by addition of sodium metabisulphite; and the U.S.P. has *Epinephrine Injection*, a sterile, 1 in 1,000, solution of the hydrochloride. For other purposes both pharmacopoeias have a non-sterilized, 1 in 1,000, *Solution of Adrenaline Hydrochloride*, B.P., *Epinephrine Solution*, U.S.P., and the U.S.P. has also an Inhalation.

For hypodermic or intramuscular use the usual dose is 0·12–0·5 ml. (2–8 min.) of the Injection. For intravenous injection the dose is much smaller, 0·06–0·12 ml. (1–2 min.), which must be well diluted with sterile saline solution and injected very slowly.

NORADRENALINE (LEVARTERENOL)

The transmitter at adrenergic nerve-ends is chiefly, if not universally, noradrenaline. In the synthesis of adrenaline in the body, noradrenaline is a precursor. The final stage in that synthesis, the methylation of nitrogen, takes place in the adrenals. This methylation may not be complete, in which case the secretion from the adrenals is a mixture of the two compounds, adrenaline predominating. Broadly speaking, the main function of noradrenaline is to produce localized effects at sympathetic nerve-ends. Adrenaline, on the other hand, is a specific hormone especially discharged into the blood to serve emergency purposes, producing generalized effects which put the animal in a condition to withstand danger (Cannon's theory), such effects including increased cardiac output, increased blood flow through the muscles and brain at the expense of the viscera and skin, possibly widening of the calibre of the bronchi to facilitate respiration.

Different species of animals vary considerably in their responses to both amines. Noradrenaline is, on injection into laboratory mammals, less toxic than adrenaline and is relatively less potent in producing inhibitory effects (e.g. relaxation of bronchi or inhibition of the rat's uterus) than motor effects (e.g. contraction of arterioles). Most investigators agree that with therapeutic doses in man, the pressor effect of noradrenaline is accompanied by an almost parallel rise in systolic and diastolic pressures with little or no change in the minute-volume of the heart; with adrenaline, however, the rise is mainly in systolic pressure and the minute-volume of the heart is increased. It would seem that, in such doses, the pressor effect of noradrenaline is due mainly to a generalized vasoconstriction, that of adrenaline mainly to an increase in cardiac output.

Noradrenaline acid tartrate, *Levarterenol Bitartrate*, U.S.P., 5 mcg. (micrograms) per minute has been used successfully in cases of serious low blood pressure due to peripheral vascular failure, such as acute hypotension following the use of ganglionic blocking agents, cardiac infarction (where there is a risk of ventricular fibrillation with adrenaline), hypotension during spinal analgesia or following sympathectomy. It should be given in a slow infusion well diluted and the patient's blood pressure checked frequently. Adrenaline would seem to be preferable in cases where failure of the circulation is due to depression of the heart muscle, e.g. in attempts to revive the heart after stoppage due to overdose of some anaesthetics. Perhaps a mixture of the two hormones might be preferable in some conditions. After all the adrenals secrete such a mixture and by this time they ought to know their business.

OTHER RELATED AMINES

Adrenaline may be regarded as a derivative of phenylethylamine, $C_6H_5CH_2CH_2NH_2$, and a glance at the constitutional formula of adrenaline will show that a vast number of compounds are possible by simple substitutions in either the catechol nucleus or the side chain, while preserving the basic conformation of phenylethylamine. Many such compounds were investigated in the pioneer and revealing work of Barger and Dale (1910). Many more have since been investigated, mostly with a view to finding superior substitutes for the various therapeutic uses of adrenaline. If they act like adrenaline, they may be called 'sympathomimetic', but few, if any, of them reproduce all the effects of sympathetic stimulation with the same fidelity as adrenaline. Of the large number of compounds that have been investigated, only those will be mentioned which have shown definite therapeutic value.

ISOPRENALINE (ISOPROTERENOL)

Isoprenaline differs from adrenaline in the substitution of an *iso*propyl group for the methyl group attached to the nitrogen. It possesses in an enhanced degree those actions of adrenaline (especially dilatation of the bronchi and increase in cardiac output) which are less conspicuously displayed by noradrenaline. It is chiefly used as **Isoprenaline Sulphate**, B.P., 5–20 mg., or **Isoproterenol Hydrochloride**, U.S.P., in asthma, and has the advantage of being effective when given orally. It may be given as tablets, sublingually, or, for rapid action, by inhalation from a solution in an atomizer, alone, or combined with other drugs.

Mephentermine Sulfate, U.S.P., (trimethylphenylethylamine), is used as a vasoconstrictor for topical application to congested nasal mucosae.

EPHEDRINE

Ephedrine, an alkaloid obtained from Ma Huang, a drug which has long been in use in China, has the formula:

$$C_6H_5 \cdot CHOH \cdot CHCH_3 \cdot NHCH_3.$$

Ephedrine possesses a much more stable molecule than adrenaline, with the following important consequences. Ephedrine is much less liable than adrenaline to chemical change as the result of exposure to light and air. It is also less affected by digestive processes and can produce systemic effects when given by mouth. It is less rapidly destroyed by the tissues, and therefore its effects are more persistent than those of adrenaline. It resembles adrenaline in action but, being less active, has to be given in much higher doses. It has the great advantage over adrenaline that it can produce its effects when given by mouth. It has a stimulant action on the central nervous system. It has been found useful especially in asthma (for dilating the bronchi), and in coryza and hay-fever in which it causes shrinkage of the nasal mucous membrane. It has a beneficial effect in some cases of myasthenia gravis, owing to a facilitating action on the nerve-ends of voluntary muscle. Owing to the rather long pressor effect, it must be given with caution to patients with cardiovascular disease. Among the disagreeable effects that may occur with overdosage may be mentioned nausea, headache, palpitation, insomnia, and retention of urine. It may be given as *Ephedrine Hydrochloride*, B.P., 16–60 mg. ($\frac{1}{4}$–1 gr.); *Ephedrine Sulfate*, U.S.P., 25–50 mg.

AMPHETAMINE

Amphetamine $C_6H_5 \cdot CH_2CH(CH_3) \cdot NH_2$, is a volatile base and was introduced as a nasal inhalant for constricting the mucous membrane in coryza, &c. Unlike adrenaline it is a powerful stimulant of the central nervous system, an action possessed to a less extent by ephedrine. In man it produces euphoria, increased wakefulness, and other symptoms of cerebral stimulation. The effects vary considerably in different persons. Therapeutically it has been used in conditions of mental depression, narcolepsy, Parkinsonism, and as an analeptic (p. 80). It is official as *Amphetamine Sulphate*, B.P., U.S.P., 2·5–10 mg.

Dexamphetamine. The dextro-isomer of amphetamine, which is a racemic compound, is dexamphetamine. It is official as *Dextro Amphetamine Sulfate* in the U.S.P. It has been much used as dexamphetamine sulphate (Dexedrine) 2·5–5 mg. for reducing obesity, an effect produced also by amphetamine sulphate. This it does chiefly by reducing gastric motility and lessening appetite, but the cerebral stimulation may help by fortifying the patient against the rigours of dieting. It is contraindicated in patients with marked hypertension, thyrotoxicosis, or insomnia.

Methylamphetamine Hydrochloride, B.P., *Methamphetamine Hydrochloride*, U.S.P., a desoxyephedrine, acts very like amphetamine. It has been used chiefly in the treatment of obesity, dose 2·5–10 mg., and as an Injection of 10–30 mg. for combating serious hypotension, e.g. following spinal anaesthesia or in narcotic poisoning. *Hydroxyamphetamine Hydrobromide*, U.S.P., is used in a 0·25–1 per cent. solution for topical application to inflamed mucosae.

Methoxamine Hydrochloride, U.S.P., dose 15 mg. intramuscularly, is a derivative of *iso*propylamine as is amphetamine but differs from the latter in having little or no stimulant effect on the central nervous system. It causes a rise in blood pressure which is well sustained and is used for this purpose in the resuscitation of patients who are suffering from circulatory failure. Unlike the more closely sympathomimetic compounds, it tends to slow the pulse rather than increase its rate.

II. *DEPRESSANTS*

There are no anti-adrenaline compounds in everyday clinical use on a scale comparable with the use of atropine or curariform drugs in relation to acetylcholine. This may in part be due to the fact that the indications for the use of such substances are not clear. It is not certain that hypertension, even in its early stages, is due to overactivity of the adrenergic vasoconstrictor nerves though lowering sympathetic tone, e.g. by ganglion block, may help the patient greatly. There are a number of diseases characterized by poor circulation in the limbs. This may be due to intermittent overactivity of the regional sympathetic nerves, as in some cases of Raynaud's disease, and will benefit from an agent which will antagonize that activity, but it may be due to mechanical closure of the vessels. There is, however, one clear indication for the use of these substances and that is the presence of a phaeochromocytoma (or adrenal medullary tumour) which produces excessive quantities of adrenaline and noradrenaline. The radical treatment is by surgical excision but the effect of an adrenaline-antagonist in producing a temporary sharp fall in blood pressure is an aid to diagnosis and these drugs may be of value during the operation. These substances antagonize the effects of injected noradrenaline less than those of adrenaline, and have least action of all on the effects of sympathetic nerve activity. If successful they inevitably give rise to postural hypotension, and other side-effects are common.

They may be classified as being of vegetable or synthetic

origin. Among the former are certain alkaloids of ergot (p. 177) and yohimbine. These are weak and the action is reversible. Among the synthetics may be mentioned *Tolazoline Hydrochloride*, U.S.P., dose 50–75 mg., which exerts direct dilating effects on the vessels of an acetylcholine-like and also a histamine-like type and in addition antagonizes adrenaline-noradrenaline to a feeble extent. It, or derivatives of it such as *Phentolamine Hydrochloride*, U.S.P., 50 mg., orally, or *Phentolamine Methanesulfonate*, U.S.P., 5 mg., by injection, are of some value in conditions of functional spasm of vessels but give rise to unpleasantly violent action of the heart due to an atropine-like activity which blocks the vagus nerve.

These and other compounds are short-acting and the effect which they produce is in proportion to the amount which is administered, i.e. their action is a competitive one. In contrast Dibenyline has a prolonged action which, once established, is independent of the dosage.

None of these 'adrenaline antagonists' does in fact antagonize all the actions of adrenaline and noradrenaline or of stimulation of adrenergic nerves. Only the 'motor' activities are affected, e.g. constriction of blood vessels and contraction of certain involuntary muscles; there is neither relaxation of smooth muscle, e.g. in the intestine, or bronchus, nor stimulation of the heart. Their uses are inevitably restricted.

XIV

DRUGS ACTING DIRECTLY ON INVOLUNTARY MUSCLE

I. *STIMULANTS*

As has already been seen, certain kinds of involuntary muscle can be stimulated to increased contraction by means of drugs which act on the autonomic nervous system; but many substances stimulate the contractions of smooth muscle by a direct action on the muscle fibre, independently of the nerve supply.

Barium salts act in this way, if soluble, but they stimulate all kinds of smooth muscle (e.g. of the blood vessels, bronchi, gut, ureter, heart, &c.) so indiscriminately that they are of little or no therapeutic value. A soluble salt like barium chloride is so highly poisonous that even a teaspoonful may prove fatal when given by mouth. ***Barium Sulphate***, B.P., U.S.P., however, is quite insoluble, and only traces can be rendered soluble in the alimentary canal. It is, therefore, non-toxic when given by mouth, and is widely used to give a shadow in X-ray examination of the alimentary canal. As it may be given in large doses for this purpose, it must be free from other barium salts.

ERGOT

Ergot is a parasitic fungus (*Claviceps purpurea*) which grows on the ovary of the rye or on other kinds of grain. As the result of this growth, the rye grains become swollen and purplish in colour. Bread made from rye thus infected has occasionally given rise to epidemics of chronic poisoning, in some of which gangrene of the fingers or toes has been a prominent feature. In other epidemics cramps and convulsions have been the main symptoms. Abortion sometimes occurs in pregnant women. This latter effect has possibly suggested the medicinal use of ergot, which began to be regularly used in obstetrics about the middle of the nineteenth century.

ERGOMETRINE

Many active substances have been found in ergot in varying amounts. From the therapeutic point of view the most important active principle is ergometrine which is chiefly responsible for the contractions of the uterus which occur when preparations like the Liquid Extract are given by mouth. It acts more rapidly than the other active principles, ergotoxine and ergotamine. Its chief action is to stimulate contractions of the uterus, especially of the puerperal uterus. It is readily soluble in water and rapidly absorbed from the alimentary canal, and when given by mouth may cause powerful and prolonged contractions of the uterus within about five minutes. It arrests post-partum haemorrhage mainly by the occlusion of the blood vessels caused by the outside pressure of the contracting uterine muscle.

It has little direct vasoconstrictor action and does not cause gangrene, nor does it antagonize adrenaline. It is therefore free from most of the toxic effects of the other alkaloids. It is especially suitable for intravenous injection, quickly arresting uterine haemorrhage after childbirth, for which purpose it has largely replaced preparations of pituitary gland.

In the U.S.P. Ergometrine is called *Ergonovine*. Dosage of *Ergometrine Maleate*, B.P., orally 0·5–1 mg.; intramuscularly, 0·25–1 mg.; intravenously, 0·125–0·5 mg. *Ergonovine Maleate*, U.S.P., oral, intramuscular, and subcutaneous, 0·2 mg.

Methylergometrine very closely resembles the parent alkaloid ergometrine and is given in similar doses. It is more soluble and may be absorbed more quickly when given orally. It also seems to have a quicker, stronger, and more lasting action on the uterus than ergometrine itself, and to be more stable.

Other important alkaloids are ergotoxine and ergotamine, which occur in different proportions in different samples of ergot. They are closely related chemically and have almost identical pharmacological actions so that they can be discussed together. They stimulate the uterine muscle, but only after a considerable latent period, even when given intravenously. They are less soluble in water than ergometrine and less active when given by mouth. They can in overdosage produce gangrene. They stimulate other forms of smooth muscle, especially of the arterioles, and cause a rise of blood pressure. They have another action of interest in connexion with the sympathetic nervous system. In larger doses they antagonize the actions, especially the motor effects, of adrenaline or of sympathetic stimulation, or may even reverse the action of adrenaline. The exact site of their action is uncertain. They do not prevent the liberation of adrenaline from the nerve-endings when a sympathetic nerve is stimulated.

Ergotamine has been widely used for the relief of migraine and other severe headaches, possibly because the dilatation of the cranial vessels, which is the cause of some headaches, is counteracted by ergotamine. It acts most effectively by injection though oral administration suffices in some cases. It must be given with care as symptoms of ergotism may occur, e.g. numbness or sensory disturbances of the skin or even gangrene, most commonly of the fingers or toes.

Ergotamine Tartrate is official in both pharmacopoeias. Single dose: B.P., orally 1–2 mg., subcutaneously or intramuscularly 0·25–0·5 mg.; U.S.P., orally 2 mg., intramuscularly 0·25 mg.

PITUITARY GLAND (POSTERIOR LOBE)

The actions of extracts of the *posterior lobe* of the pituitary gland will be considered here. It was discovered in 1895 that this extract raises blood pressure when injected intravenously. Further researches showed that the action of pituitary, unlike that of adrenaline, has no relation to nerve supply but is generally a stimulant one on smooth muscle. Its action differs, however, from that of barium in being less generalized. It seems to act most strongly on the muscle of the arterioles, uterus, and intestine, and it is for its action on these structures that it is chiefly used.

When pituitary extract is injected intravenously, it produces a rise of blood pressure which is due to constriction of the arterioles. This pressor effect is more prolonged than that of adrenaline, which it superficially resembles. Pituitary constricts the vessels of an isolated organ when perfused through them. Its action is therefore independent of the vasomotor centre; it acts, like adrenaline, peripherally. The constriction of vessels produced by pituitary bears, however, no relation to their innervation. Thus it constricts the coronary and lung vessels, whereas these, not supplied with constrictor sympathetic nerves, are unaffected by adrenaline. Pituitary is believed to act directly on the muscle of the vessels. Similarly, pituitary has no action on the isolated heart corresponding to sympathetic stimulation; indeed, what slight effect it exerts is in the direction of slowing the heart.

Pituitary has been widely used to stimulate the contractions of the uterus after labour, especially in prevention or treatment of post-partum haemorrhage but is now largely replaced by ergometrine which has fewer undesirable effects. When the placenta separates from the uterus, it leaves the connecting vessels open, and bleeding is stopped in the first instance not so much by contractions of the vessels or clotting inside them as by contraction of the muscle of the uterus itself, which occludes the vessels by pressure from without. Here speed of action is imperative, and pituitary, when injected intramuscularly, acts almost at once. Pituitary acts directly on the uterine muscle. Its stimulant action is slight in early pregnancy and increases to a maximum at parturition. It has no action when given by mouth.

Pituitary also to a less degree stimulates the movements of the gut, and is sometimes used for this purpose.

When injected intravenously in an anaesthetized animal, pituitary usually increases the secretion of urine, a transient and therapeutically unimportant effect secondary to the pressor action. Otherwise, and especially in cases of diabetes insipidus, it greatly diminishes the secretion of urine due to the presence in the extract of the antidiuretic hormone (p. 24), which checks the reabsorption of fluid from the kidney tubules.

It is now known that there are in the posterior lobe of the gland at least two active principles, which can be obtained partially separated, one mainly responsible for the action on the uterus (oxytocic), and the other for the action on the blood pressure (pressor). The antidiuretic principle is associated with the latter, but may be distinct from it. Preparations containing the active principles so separated are now in the B.P. and U.S.P. In the B.P. they have replaced the original Injection of Posterior Pituitary.

Injection of Oxytocin, B.P., U.S.P., is a sterile aqueous solution containing the oxytocic principle, prepared by a process of fractionation from the posterior lobe of the pituitary bodies of oxen and other animals. It is biologically standardized. It is used for its action on the uterus, for checking post-partum haemorrhage, or for inducing labour in toxaemia. Dose: B.P., by subcutaneous or intramuscular injection, 0·25–0·5 ml. (3–8 min.), equivalent to 2–5 Units; U.S.P., 1 ml. (10 Units). The active principle is a polypeptide, which has recently been synthesized.

Injection of Vasopressin, B.P., U.S.P., is a similar type of solution containing the pressor and antidiuretic principles. It also stimulates uterine contractions, especially and unlike oxytocin in early pregnancy, and may be used to control haemorrhage occurring after early abortion. Its chief uses are in diabetes insipidus for the action of its antidiuretic hormone (p. 24), to stimulate the muscle of the gut in cases of atony, and to raise blood pressure in some cases of shock. Dose: B.P., by subcutaneous or intramuscular injection, 0·25–0·75 ml. (4–12 min.), equivalent to 5–15 Units; U.S.P., 1 ml.

The *anterior lobe* of the pituitary contains several hormones which will be discussed later (p. 223).

HISTAMINE

Adrenaline, noradrenaline, acetylcholine, and histamine form a quarto of compounds found in the body and capable of producing effects in extremely low concentrations. The normal functions of the first three have already been considered, that of histamine is still obscure. The complicated actions of histamine would necessitate little consideration here in so far as it is of therapeutic value, but in certain conditions in man toxic effects are produced by the liberation of histamine, and the positive effects of antihistamine compounds, later to be discussed, are due to the suppression of these toxic effects.

Histamine has three main actions:

(i) It is a general stimulant of almost all plain muscle, but its action varies quantitatively in different muscles and in different species of animals. It stimulates uterine muscle in most animals and may cause severe broncho-constriction especially in guinea-pigs.

(ii) It causes dilatation of the capillaries. Effects on blood pressure vary in different animals depending on the relative degree of action on the arterioles and on the capillaries. In most animals, including man, capillary dilatation predominates; there may be a profound fall of blood pressure and fluid escapes from the dilated capillaries, with a consequent increased concentration of the plasma (vascular shock). A threefold reaction, shown by Lewis, results from pricking histamine into the skin—local redness, oedema, and a surrounding arterial dilatation.

Similar effects occur from the sting of the nettle (*urtica*), the hairs of which contain histamine, and in an allergic reaction in man the skin effects (more or less widely diffused) are so similar that the condition has been called urticaria.

(iii) Histamine increases the secretion from many glands, e.g. salivary, intestinal, and lachrymal, and especially from the gastric glands.

Most tissues, including blood, contain histamine but in the cells it is mostly held in an inactive state owing to some form of combination. In allergy the symptoms are believed to be due to the release of histamine in an active form due to a disturbance of the colloidal suspension of the protoplasm, and the symptoms reproduce more or fewer of the effects of histamine according to the causal factor and the particular tissues involved. Of the symptoms, only one of which may occur in an individual, the most important are: asthma, due to broncho-constriction; urticaria; irritation of mucous membranes, e.g.

of the nose in hay-fever; gastro-intestinal disturbances, or a fall in blood pressure. Allergy is usually due to sensitization of a person to some protein, e.g. in pollens or in certain foods, but may also occur with certain drugs.

Histamine is produced in the body by decarboxylation of the amino-acid histidine and inactivated by an enzyme, histaminase. Large amounts of histamine are present in the intestine but are not normally absorbed into the blood in an active form, partly because some of it is acetylated by bacteria and so inactivated, and partly because the mucous membrane of the intestine contains much histaminase which hydrolyses histamine.

Histamine consequently produces little effect when swallowed and is accordingly administered subcutaneously as *Injection of Histamine Acid Phosphate*, B.P., U.S.P., 1 mg. in 1 ml.; dose: B.P. 0·5–1 mg.; U.S.P., 0·3 mg., as a test for the presence of functioning gastric mucosa.

ANTIHISTAMINES

Although not muscle stimulants, the antihistamines can be most conveniently considered in relation to histamine. Once it was realized that many disabilities result from the abnormal release of histamine in the body, search was begun for drugs which could antagonize its action. No antagonist has been found among natural plant alkaloids but, during the last decade or more, a lengthy and still growing list of synthetic antagonists has been discovered, only a few of which can be mentioned here. Some of them resemble, but not always very closely, histamine in structure, and apparently act by blocking the tissue receptors for histamine, without actually lessening its liberation. Generally these drugs find their main clinical use in allergic conditions of the skin and mucous membranes. They have often a dramatic effect in relieving urticaria, including that produced by antibiotics, and angioneurotic oedema. In hay-fever and perennial vasomotor rhinitis, the sneezing and rhinorrhoea are checked in a high proportion of cases. They have little effect in common colds, which are due to a virus infection. They have given disappointing results in spasmodic asthma or anaphylaxis, possibly because in these conditions histamine is released within the cells and beyond reach of the drugs in the blood. They do not antagonize the stimulating action of histamine on the gastric secretion.

Certain toxic or side-effects are common to most of them. Drowsiness is a usual reaction, often lessening with continued use. This is due to a depressant action on the central nervous system similar to that produced by hyoscine. Use is made of this action in the treatment of travel sickness (p. 115) and in Parkinsonism (p. 113). Many of them have additional pharmacological actions, e.g. local anaesthetic or atropine-like. The latter action probably accounts for the dryness of the mouth which is a common side-effect.

All the antihistamines can be given by mouth, as they are absorbed from the intestine. They vary in the speed, intensity, and duration of action. They do not effect a permanent cure, as the underlying allergic tendency persists.

The following are official or widely used. There are at present too many of these compounds available in view of the relatively small part which they play in therapeutics and it is desirable to get to know the actions of one or two.

Mepyramine Maleate, B.P., dose 0·3–0·8 G. per day, *Pyrilamine Maleate*, U.S.P., dose 100 mg. per day, is quick, powerful, and relatively short-lasting. It may cause drowsiness and dizziness.

Promethazine Hydrochloride, B.P., dose 25–75 mg. per day, is structurally related to Ethopropazine and Chlorpromazine (p. 110). It is slow to act, powerful, and long-lasting. It causes drowsiness. *Diphenhydramine Hydrochloride*, U.S.P., dose 50 mg., is rapid in onset, short-lasting, powerful, and a potent hypnotic. *Dimenhydrinate*, U.S.P., is the name given to a compound of the above with *Theophylline* (p. 80) which is much used for the control of motion sickness. *Tripelennamine Hydrochloride*, U.S.P., dose 50 mg., is closely related to Mepyramine (Pyrilamine) and has almost identical properties. *Antazoline Hydrochloride*, U.S.P., is related to Tolazoline. It is used mainly for topical application as a solution to the nasal membranes in allergic rhinitis. A cream for application to itching areas of skin exerts a double action—antihistamine and local anaesthetic. *Chlorcyclizine Hydrochloride*, U.S.P., dose 50 mg., has a very prolonged action. *Chlorpheniramine Maleate*, U.S.P., dose 4 mg., is a compound of outstanding potency. The low dosage ensures relative freedom from side effects. *Chlorothen Citrate*, U.S.P., dose 25 mg., and *Thonzylamine Hydrochloride*, U.S.P., dose 50 mg., are effective and produce less depression than some others. *Phenindamine Tartrate*, U.S.P., dose 25 mg., is a stimulant of the central nervous system and may be used in combination with or as an alternative to the others.

II. DEPRESSANTS

NITRITES

There are various ways whereby the tone or rhythmic movements of smooth muscle can be reduced, e.g. by paralysis of motor nerve effects (atropine), by stimulation of inhibitor nerve effects (adrenaline), or by depression of smooth muscle directly, their action being unrelated to nerve supply. The nitrites, which are now to be considered, act by depressing smooth muscle directly.

As has been pointed out before in the case of stimulants of smooth muscle, it is not to be expected that nitrites will act quantitatively alike on smooth muscle in different organs. They act most vigorously on the muscle of the arterioles. They also act definitely on the muscle of the bronchi. They affect chiefly the tone of smooth muscle, and seem to have less effect in inhibiting rhythmic movements. They are therefore chiefly used for widening conduits with smooth muscle walls.

Amyl Nitrite, B.P., U.S.P., 0·12–0·3 ml. (2–5 min.) by inhalation, is a liquid, soluble in alcohol or ether but almost insoluble in water. It has a fruity odour and a pungent taste. It is administered by inhalation. When inhaled, it causes flushing of the skin, at first of the head and neck, but later of the rest of the body. This is due to the dilatation of the arterioles. Larger doses dilate also the arterioles of internal organs. Owing to the relaxation of the vessels there is a rapid fall of blood pressure. It often produces a sensation of throbbing in the head. The heart is reflexly quickened by the fall of pressure, but amyl nitrite has no direct effects of importance upon the heart. In the perfused isolated heart, for example, the coronary vessels are dilated by amyl nitrite, but the actual heart beats are hardly influenced.

This effect on the vessels is due to a direct action of amyl nitrite on their muscle walls. It occurs in perfused isolated organs, where any action on the vasomotor centre is of course excluded. Amyl nitrite has a somewhat similar action on other forms of smooth muscle, especially on that of the bronchi.

The physiological activity of amyl nitrite is due mainly to the nitrite part of the molecule, and a similar action is exerted by many other nitrites (e.g. sodium nitrite) in which the group $O \cdot NO$ is found. Inorganic nitrates (like sodium nitrate) which have the group $O \cdot NO_2$ do not possess this action, but certain *nitric esters*, such as glyceryl trinitrate, are partly reduced in the body into nitrites and have an action similar to nitrites. These nitric esters are therefore conveniently included in the group of nitrites. They similarly relax smooth muscle but differ from one another chiefly in regard to the speed and duration of action. These time-differences are of importance in determining the suitability of each for particular conditions.

THERAPEUTIC USES OF NITRITES AND NITRIC ESTERS. Amyl nitrite acts very rapidly, but its action is over in a few minutes. It was introduced by Brunton for the relief of angina pectoris, a cardiac attack characterized by sudden onset, great pain, and sometimes by a rise of blood pressure. Its beneficial effect in this condition is believed to be due largely to its dilating the coronary vessels. In angina pectoris the remedy is required at once, and for convenience and for accuracy of dose, amyl nitrite is usually put up in glass capsules which can be broken in a handkerchief and the nitrite inhaled. It is sometimes similarly given in asthma, which it relieves by relaxing the spasmodically constricted bronchi. Large doses of amyl nitrite tend to produce methaemoglobin in the blood.

Glyceryl Trinitrate (Nitroglycerin) is an explosive substance which as such is unsuited for medicinal use. It is official as special *Tablets of Glyceryl Trinitrate*, B.P., U.S.P., in which it is incorporated with a chocolate basis. Dose 0·5–1 mg. ($\frac{1}{130}$–$\frac{1}{60}$ gr.). These should be chewed and sucked, not swallowed whole, as absorption is most rapid from the buccal mucous membrane. It takes longer (a few minutes) to act than amyl nitrite but the vascular dilatation lasts longer. It is used for similar purposes but is more convenient to take. It causes severe headaches in some people.

Of other nitric esters that have been used, *Pentaerythritol Tetranitrate* is favoured for its long action and absence of side-effects.

Among other drugs which are used to relax smooth muscle may be mentioned papaverine (p. 118), volatile oils (p. 43), and aminophylline (p. 80).

XV

DRUGS ACTING ON HEART MUSCLE

WE have had numerous examples of drugs which influence the tone or rhythmic contractions of smooth muscle, either in the direction of stimulation or of depression, and produce their effects either on the muscle directly or in association with the nerve supply. We have also seen that most drugs exercise some selective action on smooth muscle; for example, pituitary stimulates the muscle of the uterus to a much greater extent than that of the bronchi, and nitrites have a more powerful dilating effect on the muscle of the arterioles than on the smooth muscle of most other organs. It is not surprising, therefore, that when we come to a type of involuntary muscle like the heart, which has diverged very considerably from the usual type of smooth muscle, this selective action will be even more apparent. For example, pituitary and nitrites have hardly any direct effect on heart muscle at all. Conversely, it would be reasonable to expect that some drugs would influence the contractions of the heart, while having relatively little effect on other forms of involuntary muscle, and this is true of one very important group of therapeutic agents, sometimes called the cardiac tonics, which, at least in the case of smaller doses, have a powerful action on the heart while exercising little action on other forms of involuntary muscle. To this group belongs a large number of plants whose active principles all have a very similar qualitative effect on the heart. In the case of all these plants the active principles have been found to be glycosides. Of this group only two official members need be considered, digitalis and strophanthus. Of these digitalis is the more important and will be considered first. Squill which belongs to this group is no longer official.

DIGITALIS

Digitalis, the leaves of the foxglove, *Digitalis purpurea*, was introduced into regular medicine by the distinguished physician and scientist William Withering, who in 1785 published a book advocating its use as a diuretic, based upon a clinical experience extending over the previous ten years. It was not fully realized until long afterwards that this diuretic effect produced by digitalis is the result of an improvement in the blood supply of the kidney, and consequent upon an action of the digitalis not upon the kidney directly but upon the heart. Digitalis has gradually attained a place of the first importance in the treatment of diseases of the heart.

ACTION ON THE HEART. The full story of the actions on the heart cannot be told here. The actions differ according to the species of animal, and in the same animal under different conditions of cardiac disease. Here it is only possible to give an elementary account of those actions in so far as they subserve the therapeutic uses of digitalis in man. It has been known for half a century or more that, in many cases of cardiac disease accompanied by undue rapidity and by irregularity of the heart beats, digitalis can slow the pulse, improve the circulation, and remove symptoms, such as oedema, defective secretion of urine, &c., which are the result of the impairment of the circulation. Especially in the last half-century, a large number of researches have been devoted to obtaining a more precise delimitation of the varieties of cardiac disease in which digitalis can be effectively employed and towards a more accurate explanation of its method of action.

Digitalis has three important actions on the heart. By a direct action on the myocardium it: (i) increases the force of contraction and (ii) prolongs the refractory period; by stimulating the vagus centre it (iii) slows the heart.

Digitalis in the first place increases the force of the contraction of the heart. In the initial stage this is shown by a slight increase and prolongation of ventricular systole. If the concentration be increased, the systole is prolonged and the relaxation diminished until the heart stops in systole. This is the most characteristic action of the glycosides of the digitalis group.

The slowing of the heart by digitalis may be brought about in different ways. In the normal heart it is mainly due to stimulation of the vagus centre. Thus in the mammal it does not occur in the normal perfused isolated heart, and in the intact animal is prevented by atropine. A supplementary and important cause of the slowing produced by digitalis in cardiac disease has more recently been emphasized. In the condition known as auricular fibrillation, digitalis may slow the heart in spite of the simultaneous administration of atropine; in this case the slowing cannot be due to stimulation of the vagus centre, for atropine would prevent these stimuli reaching the heart. It has been found that in auricular fibrillation digitalis slows the pulse by lengthening the refractory period of the heart muscle. When the auricle is fibrillating, the ventricle is bombarded by rapid feeble impulses from the auricle, and responds by beating as fast as it can, and the beats have no regularity. Digitalis by this second action prevents a great number of these impulses from reaching the ventricle and so the heart-rate is slowed, though the fibrillation of the auricle is not necessarily, or usually, stopped by digitalis.

If the dose is sufficiently large, the conduction through the auriculo-ventricular bundle may be so diminished that complete heart block results, the ventricle beating independently with its own slow rhythm.

In auricular flutter, a condition in which the auricle contracts (with a sort of circus movement) regularly but very fast and the ventricle responds by a rapid regular rhythm, digitalis in many cases first changes the auricular flutter into fibrillation, which in turn may disappear and be replaced by normal rhythm when the digitalis administration is discontinued.

Quinidine (p. 194) is also used in the treatment of auricular fibrillation and flutter.

In cases of heart disease when the heart is beating very rapidly and irregularly, the output of the heart per unit of time is diminished. This is so because the diastolic pause is of too short duration to enable the heart to fill completely, and also because usually the contraction is too feeble to expel completely even this limited quantity of blood. By prolonging the diastolic pause digitalis allows the heart to fill more completely, and by augmenting the force of systole it enables the heart to empty itself more completely. The output per unit of time is increased in spite of the slowing, and the velocity of the peripheral circulation can be shown to be greater. More blood is driven into the arteries and the congestion of the veins is relieved. The condition of the heart itself is improved by the increase in its own blood- (and therefore oxygen-) supply.

All organs of the body suffer if the circulation is defective. This is conspicuously so in the case of the kidney. In many cases of heart disease there may be, owing to impairment of the blood flow through the kidney, a marked diminution in the secretion of urine and widespread oedema of the body. In these cases digitalis, by improving the circulation through the kidney, often produces an enormous increase in the flow of urine and a rapid removal of the oedema. It was for this diuretic effect that Withering first used it. It must be remembered that this diuretic action is not a direct one on the kidney. It does not occur, for example, in animals with a normal circulation. It is an effect secondary to improvement of the circulation where that is defective. In practice the diuretic action of digitalis is often supplemented by a mercurial or other diuretic, to accelerate the removal of oedema fluid.

This increase in the output of the heart is by far the most important action of digitalis, and indeed, in small doses, almost its only action. Higher concentrations than are required to produce a therapeutic effect on the heart may act on involuntary muscle in other organs, for example on the muscle of the arterioles or uterus; but these effects are not likely to be produced by medicinal doses of digitalis in man.

The digitalis glycosides are irritating substances and may produce nausea and vomiting, both by irritation of the stomach as well as by an action on the vomiting centre which, like the cardiac vagus centre, they stimulate. The glycosides are slowly absorbed from the alimentary canal, so that, when given in the ordinary way by mouth, digitalis usually takes two or three days to produce its full effect. They are also slowly eliminated, so that, once the effect on the heart is produced, it usually persists for several days after digitalis is discontinued.

CUMULATION. The rate of elimination may be even slower than that of absorption, so that, if given continuously, digitalis may accumulate in the body and its action go beyond what is intended or desirable. Symptoms of cumulative overdosage produced in this way are headache, nausea, and vomiting; undue slowing of the heart, sometimes with pulsus bigeminus; extrasystoles; diminution of urinary secretion; occasionally the heart may stop from ventricular fibrillation. Recognition of the early toxic symptoms is important because for fully effective digitalization the doses required are not far short of toxic doses.

As there is no known convenient method of chemically assaying preparations of digitalis, these have to be standardized by some pharmacological test, the activity of the preparation to be tested being compared with that of a standard preparation of digitalis. The criterion of activity used for this comparison may be the amount required to produce systolic arrest of the heart of the frog when the preparations are injected into a lymph-sac, or the amount required to arrest the heart of the cat when the preparations are injected intravenously. Whatever be the biological method employed, groups of animals are necessary for such a comparison, partly to eliminate individual variations in susceptibility.

Several preparations of digitalis leaf and some of the glycosidal active principles are used medicinally. They all produce similar effects on the heart and circulation but differ in their degree of absorption and in speed and duration of effect.

PREPARATIONS OF DIGITALIS. In the B.P. the unstandardized Digitalis Leaf (the leaves of the common purple-flowered foxglove *Digitalis purpurea*) is used only for making preparations. For medicinal use there are three standardized preparations: **Prepared Digitalis**, B.P. (1 Unit in 0·1 G.), 30–100 mg.,

($\frac{1}{2}$–1$\frac{1}{2}$ gr.); *Tablets of Prepared Digitalis*, 30–100 mg. ($\frac{1}{2}$–1$\frac{1}{2}$ gr.); *Tincture of Digitalis* (1 Unit in 1 ml.), 0·3–1 ml. (5–15 min.). The maximum dose of each preparation contains one Unit of activity. Owing to its poor keeping qualities the tincture is much less used now than formerly and may soon be abandoned. The Tablets are the most frequently prescribed preparation of digitalis in this country. The U.S.P. has *Powdered Digitalis*, 100 mg. daily; *Digitalis Tablets*, 100 mg., and *Digitalis Capsules*, 100 mg.

ACTIVE PRINCIPLES OF DIGITALIS. The glycosidal active principles of digitalis are difficult to isolate pure and are unstable, especially in solution. They are usually soluble in alcohol but sparingly, if at all, in water. They have a very complex structure and usually break up on hydrolysis into 'genins', which have a sterol nucleus, and sugars, some of which are peculiar to these glycosides. Somewhat different glycosides occur in two species of digitalis, *D. purpurea* and *D. lanata*.

Digitoxin. There is present in both these species a glycoside called digitoxin which is difficult to extract in pure form. This substance is absorbed and excreted very slowly and is often used for maintenance therapy, i.e. to keep the patient's cardiac muscle under the continuing influence of non-toxic amounts of digitalis for the remainder of life, once the more urgent task of restoring compensation, strengthening the failing muscle, and relieving shortness of breath and dropsy has been accomplished. It is official in the U.S.P. (maintenance dose 0·1 mg. per day), which may be given as Tablet or Injection. Being relatively impure it has to be standardized.

Digoxin, B.P., U.S.P. In *Digitalis lanata* there is found a glycoside digoxin which is relatively easy to extract in pure form, so that it may be dispensed by weight. It is almost insoluble in water, more soluble in alcohol and is absorbed from the intestine and excreted in the urine more rapidly than the glycosides of *Digitalis purpurea*, from which plant it is absent. As a result it exerts its action more speedily when given by mouth; it may be given slowly by intravenous injection in emergency (having largely replaced injection of ouabain for this purpose), and the patient will recover more quickly from inadvertent overdosage. These advantages have led to its gradually replacing the older preparations of digitalis leaf. For oral administration it is usually given as **Tablets of Digoxin**, B.P., initial dose 1–1·5 mg., maintenance dose 0·25 mg. once or twice daily; **Digoxin Tablets**, U.S.P., initial dose 1·5 mg., maintenance dose, 0·5 mg. daily. For intravenous use there is a special **Injection of Digoxin**, B.P., **Digoxin Injection**, U.S.P., for which an alcoholic solution is mixed immediately before use with saline solution; dose: B.P., 10–20 ml. (0·5–1 mg. of digoxin); U.S.P., 4 ml. (containing 1 mg.).

The close similarity of the names Digitoxin and Digoxin may lead to confusion. They must be carefully distinguished.

STROPHANTHUS

The seeds of various species of strophanthus have been used by natives of Africa for the preparation of arrow poisons. These arrow poisons were investigated, over half a century ago, by Fraser, who found that strophanthus had actions on the heart similar to those of digitalis and recommended it as a substitute for the latter in the treatment of heart disease.

The actions and uses of strophanthus are so similar to those of digitalis that they need not be recapitulated. For oral administration, digitalis is usually and deservedly preferred to strophanthus, preparations of which are no longer official.

From one species of strophanthus (*S. gratus*) a crystalline glycoside can be obtained—**Ouabain**, B.P., (Strophanthin-G), which is soluble about 1 per cent. in water and does not require biological standardization. This can be used when a rapid action on the heart is necessary. As it is a very powerful poison in overdosage, great caution is needed with regard to dose and rate of injection. It is given by slow intravenous injection, **Injection of Ouabain**, B.P., 0·12–0·25 mg.; **Ouabain Injection**, U.S.P., up to 0·5 mg., usually dissolved in 10–20 ml. of sterile water or saline. A decrease in heart rate may occur in half an hour and a full effect in 6 hours.

QUINIDINE

Quinidine, a dextro-rotatory isomer of quinine, has much the same action and activity as quinine itself. It is used chiefly in the treatment of auricular fibrillation. It was noticed that, in patients who suffered from both malaria and auricular fibrillation, quinine sometimes stopped the fibrillation of the auricle. Quinidine was found more effective for this purpose. It does not act in the same way as digitalis (p. 188), but by prolonging the refractory period of the auricular muscle. In many cases quinidine restores the normal rhythm, whereas digitalis usually slows the ventricular rate without abolishing the fibrillation of the auricle. The sudden restoration of normal auricular beats by quinidine may dislodge a clot from the auricle and when the possibility of this occurrence is suspected digitalis is safer. Quinidine must therefore be given with caution. Usually a preliminary dose is given to see whether the patient is unduly sensitive to it. The official preparation is *Quinidine Sulphate*, B.P., 60–300 mg. (1–5 gr.); U.S.P., 200–400 mg.

XVI

DRUGS ACTING ON THE RESPIRATORY SYSTEM

RESPIRATION, so far as absorption of oxygen and elimination of carbon dioxide in the lungs are concerned, is so finely regulated that, unless under very abnormal conditions, it can safely be left to itself. The respiratory centre can be excited either by excess of carbonic acid, or less directly by lack of oxygen, in the blood, the former factor being under ordinary conditions by far the more important. Defective ventilation in the lungs, therefore, which is sufficient to cause a rise of CO_2 in the blood stimulates the respiratory centre via the carotid body chemoreceptors and directly; this increases the depth of the respiratory movements and so increases the elimination of CO_2 from the blood, which in turn removes the abnormal stimulus to the respiratory centre. Under ordinary physiological conditions the elimination of carbon dioxide, and incidentally the supply of oxygen to the tissues, is thus automatically regulated.

OXYGEN

In a healthy person under normal atmospheric pressure, the tension of oxygen in the alveoli, when air is breathed, is sufficient adequately to saturate the haemoglobin of the blood passing through the lungs; and, therefore, no material increase in the oxygen-carrying capacity of the blood can be obtained by increasing the percentage of oxygen to above that already present in the air. Under certain abnormal conditions, however, the supply of oxygen to the tissues, upon which their normal functioning is so immediately dependent, may be defective. Especially in pneumonia or oedema of the lungs, oxygen may have difficulty in passing through the swollen alveolar wall. Such oxygen lack may produce, among other symptoms, hyperpnoea, cyanosis, and increased pulse rate.

In some of these conditions, e.g. in acute lobar pneumonia

or in some forms of circulatory failure, administration of oxygen in concentrations higher than the 20 per cent. in air may abolish the cyanosis and dyspnoea, lower the pulse rate, and produce a marked improvement in the subjective condition of the patient.

Oxygen, B.P., U.S.P., is stored at high pressure in steel cylinders which are coloured black with a white top bearing the name of the gas. It is difficult to devise a practical method of administering it economically and without causing discomfort to the patient. The most efficient methods of administering oxygen involve the use of a mask and valves; but many patients, already enfeebled, are unable to tolerate the mask. Oxygen can also be given to a patient enclosed in a special tent. More frequently oxygen is administered by a nasal catheter which, though less efficient, causes less discomfort. The amount of oxygen carried in solution in the plasma as a result of this administration may be sufficient to bring about improvement in conditions where the oxygen-carrying capacity of the blood is dangerously reduced, e.g. carbon monoxide poisoning. An average amount to administer is 5 litres per minute and the gas should be passed through a flask of warm water if it is to be given for long. Continued administration of high concentrations of oxygen for over 24 hours may cause an inflammation of the respiratory passages.

STIMULANTS OF THE RESPIRATORY CENTRE

The respiratory centre is exceedingly sensitive to changes in the CO_2 tension in the blood, any increase of which causes a corresponding increase in the depth, and later in the frequency, of the respiratory movements. The normal respiratory centre, therefore, finds a powerful stimulus to hand, when necessary, in the rise of tension of CO_2 in the blood. A rise of CO_2 in the inspired air from the normal of 0·04 per cent. to 2 per cent. will increase the total alveolar ventilation by as much as 50 per cent. This degree of sensitiveness of the respiratory centre to CO_2 is true, however, only if the respiratory centre be normally excitable. Like other parts of the central nervous system its excitability may be diminished by toxins or other poisons circulating in the blood. In such conditions it may be necessary to stimulate the respiratory centre. This can be done in one, or a combination, of two ways, either by augmenting the existing stimuli to the respiratory centre or by increasing the sensitiveness of the centre to stimuli already present.

A natural application of the former method is to increase the amount of **Carbon Dioxide**, B.P., U.S.P. (up to 3 per cent. or more), in the inspired air. For inhalation it is stored in grey cylinders. From the difficulties of giving it, and the dangers of too high concentration, carbon dioxide can, however, have only a limited therapeutic application. The inhalation of oxygen containing about 5–7 per cent. of Carbon Dioxide has been found valuable in the treatment of asphyxia due to drowning, carbon monoxide poisoning, and in asphyxia of the new-born. Oxygen by itself will often restore the sensitivity of the centres to the CO_2 already in the blood. When respiration is arrested the inhalation must of course be effected by some form of artificial respiration.

On the other hand the sensitiveness of the centre to stimuli already present can be heightened by the action of drugs which excite it, e.g. **Caffeine** (p. 76), Lobeline (p. 81), and **Strychnine** (p. 82). **Nikethamide** (p. 82), **Leptazol** (p. 81), **Picrotoxin** (p. 81), and **Nalorphine** (p. 121) have been used, especially in cases of narcotic poisoning.

When any or all of these measures fail, there is still left the possibility of applying artificial respiration. This is naturally of little or no enduring value in cases where the respiratory centre or lungs are irremediably damaged, as is unfortunately the case in many diseases. In cases, however, where the respiratory centre is only temporarily depressed and can recover when the causative poison is eliminated, e.g. in poisoning by narcotics or anaesthetics, artificial respiration, even though it may have to be kept up for many hours, can often save life. The newer techniques of bronchial suction and endotracheal intubation have made it possible to assist respiration with oxygen-enriched air. If necessary a mechanical respirator may be used.

DRUGS ACTING ON THE COUGH CENTRE

Pathological conditions of the air passages, especially when they give rise to cough, very frequently call for treatment. Before considering the action of drugs used in this connexion it is necessary to appreciate the mechanisms which exist for maintaining the functional integrity of the air passages themselves.

The mucous membranes of the trachea and bronchi are supplied with a wealth of mucous glands, the secretion of which keeps the surfaces moist, and can serve to dilute irritants if necessary. For removing foreign bodies, including dust and bacteria, which gain entrance into the air passages, or for removing too copious or too viscid a secretion from the bronchial mucous membrane itself, the normal mechanism is the movement of the cilia which line the inner surface of trachea and bronchi. This ciliary movement is a powerful propulsive movement which acts in effect like a moving staircase, continuously carrying up excessive secretion or foreign particles till they reach the throat and are swallowed. This mechanism is, under ordinary conditions, so quietly effective that we are unaware of its activity or even of the need of it. When, however, it becomes unable to perform the necessary scavenging, a second and reserve propulsive movement comes into play—that of cough which forcibly expels secretion or foreign particles from the interior of the air passages. Cough involves a co-ordination and timing of different muscles, and therefore necessitates a 'centre'. As the muscles involved are respiratory muscles, it is natural to find that this cough centre is intimately connected, in site and action, with the respiratory centre.

Being a purposive and useful mechanism, designed to expel material from the air passages, cough does not always necessitate treatment, and any successful effort to modify it requires skill and experience. Only the elementary considerations involved in symptomatic treatment of cough can be considered here.

Cough, though like respiration partly under voluntary

control, is usually excited reflexly, the normal stimulus being irritation of the mucous membrane of the air passages, which stimulus passes up the afferent branches of the vagus to the cough centre in the medulla. The provocative stimulus is usually accumulated secretion, but irritation of the mucous membrane to a degree sufficient to excite cough reflex may occur, for example, from a dry congestive condition of the mucous membrane when there is nothing to be coughed up. Also, stimuli of afferent branches of the vagus, other than those coming from the mucous membrane of the air passages, may, especially if prolonged, cause cough. For example, cough may be set up by irritation of the pharynx, pleura, stomach, &c. In such cases cough is useless and, as it involves considerable physical effort and may prevent sleep, it may be exhausting. It may be advantageous, therefore, to check it, and one method of doing this is to diminish the excitability of the cough centre so that the irritation ceases to excite it. The most effective remedy for this purpose is morphine or its derivatives, e.g. codeine (p. 118). Cough can sometimes be relieved by reducing afferent irritation, e.g. by inhalation of water vapour, or of menthol, which acts as a mild local anaesthetic.

DRUGS ACTING ON THE BRONCHIAL SECRETION

When the bronchial mucous membrane is in a dry and irritable condition, giving rise to cough, this can often be relieved, without the dangers attaching to morphine, merely by increasing the bronchial secretion. Also when the secretion is so viscid that it can be coughed up only with difficulty, expectoration can be facilitated by promoting a freer secretion, which will diminish the viscidity of the bronchial contents. Substances which increase bronchial secretion, called *Expectorants*, are therefore very often of use. A great many substances are known which have this action and they act in different ways. The bronchial secretion, like the salivary secretion for example, is under nervous control, and it is normally excited reflexly by stimuli from the bronchial mucous membrane. These travel up afferent branches of the vagus to the secretory centre, and are reflected down the efferent secretory branches of the vagus supplying the mucous glands.

Increased bronchial secretion can be produced by stimulation at any point of this reflex arc. On the efferent side, it can be stimulated at the centre itself. *Apomorphine Hydrochloride*, B.P., U.S.P. (p. 122), is the most important drug which stimulates the centre for bronchial secretion, but it is more often used in larger doses to excite the neighbouring vomiting centre. The receptors of the efferent secretory branches of the vagus can be stimulated, e.g. by *Pilocarpine Nitrate* (p. 156), but, as this alkaloid at the same time stimulates other vagal activities, it is difficult to obtain with it increased bronchial secretion without other simultaneous and undesirable effects. An increase of bronchial secretion can be induced also by drugs which act on the glands themselves, apart from their nerve supply. Salts, like *Potassium Iodide* (p. 205), which are excreted by the bronchial glands, act in this way, and potassium iodide will often produce a very free bronchial secretion.

Actual experience, however, has shown that the type of expectorant that is most generally useful is one which acts reflexly, that is to say, which stimulates the afferent side of the reflex arc. The normal afferent stimuli for bronchial secretion arise from irritation of the bronchial mucous membrane, and such a stimulus could be applied by administering drugs by inhalation. Apart from the difficulty of administering drugs in this way, however, it might obviously do as much harm as good if one were to apply irritants to a bronchial mucous membrane which is already in the circumstances inflamed. Fortunately, bronchial secretion, like cough, can be reflexly excited by afferent branches of the vagus other than those coming from the bronchial mucous membrane itself, especially by those coming from the gastric mucous membrane. It has in fact been found empirically that a great many drugs, which have no common pharmacological property other than that of being gastric irritants, will, when given by mouth, provoke bronchial secretion. Naturally, such gastric irritants, when given in sufficient doses, produce a degree of irritation sufficient to provoke reflex vomiting. Hence many drugs, which are used in larger doses as emetics, can be used in smaller doses as expectorants. It may be recalled that there are many muscular contractions common to the acts of vomiting and coughing (e.g. the preliminary inspiration, closure of laryngeal muscles, and contraction of the abdominal walls), so that there should be some degree of overlapping of the centre for vomiting with those for cough and bronchial secretion is not surprising.

Among the expectorants which increase bronchial secretion reflexly by irritation of the stomach may be mentioned *Ammonium Carbonate* (p. 34), *Antimony Potassium Tartrate* (p. 69), and *Ipecacuanha* (p. 30). These all possess other actions for which they are discussed elsewhere.

The drugs which have so far been discussed for their action on bronchial secretion all increase that secretion. Drugs are also known which can diminish bronchial secretion, but they are medicinally of less importance because there are fewer conditions of disease in which it is desirable to lessen the bronchial secretion. Of the drugs which have this action, *Atropine* (p. 160), and *Hyoscine* (p. 163), are the most important. They produce their effect by paralysing the secretory fibres of the vagus supplying the mucous glands, thus acting oppositely to pilocarpine. In cases of bronchitis, with a profuse watery secretion, or even in oedema of the lungs, atropine is often of value. An injection of atropine or hyoscine may also be given prior to anaesthesia, to check the profuse bronchial secretion that it is apt to produce.

DRUGS ACTING ON BRONCHIAL MUSCLE

In the previous section we have considered drugs which modify the secretion from the bronchial mucous membrane. We have now to consider an important group of drugs which alter the calibre of the bronchi. The bronchi consist of tubes with walls of smooth muscle lined by mucous membrane. The muscle of the bronchi, like smooth muscle in most organs, has a double nerve supply, motor fibres coming from the vagus (parasympathetic) nerve, and inhibitor or dilating fibres coming from the sympathetic. The vagus also, as we have seen, supplies secretory fibres to the glands of the bronchial mucous membrane, so that when the appropriate branches of the vagus nerve are stimulated, two effects are produced on the bronchi—narrowing of the calibre from contraction of the muscle, and increased secretion from stimulation of the glands.

The act of coughing, as we have seen, involves largely contractions of voluntary muscles, and is partly under voluntary control, but changes in the tonus of the involuntary muscle of the bronchi cannot be voluntarily controlled and occur without producing conscious sensations apart from effects on respiration.

Many drugs are known which can cause contraction of the bronchial muscle with resulting narrowing of the lumen of the tubes. Especially important are those which stimulate vagal activity, e.g. pilocarpine and physostigmine. By stimulating the secretory nerve-endings, these also increase bronchial secretion. The bronchi can also be constricted by substances which stimulate the muscle directly. Histamine (p. 180), acting in this way, produces, especially in herbivora, powerful constriction of the bronchi, and pituitary (p. 178) has a similar, but fortunately much feebler, action. Broncho-constrictors, as they are sometimes but inelegantly called, are, however, of little or no therapeutic importance, because few if any diseases are known in which it would be advantageous to narrow the calibre of the bronchi. It is an effect which has to be kept in mind rather with a view to its avoidance.

It is otherwise, however, with drugs which dilate the bronchi, for there are diseases in which an abnormal constriction of the bronchi occurs and in which great relief can be obtained by dilating them. Perhaps the most important of these diseases is spasmodic asthma, in attacks of which the lumen of the bronchi may be so reduced as to interfere seriously with the passage of air into and out of the lungs.

The bronchi may be dilated by drugs which act in a variety of ways, which may be more readily understood if one regards an asthmatic attack as a reflex spasm. In the first place afferent provocative stimuli may be cut off. These sometimes arise from the mucous membrane of the nose or air passages. Spraying the nose with cocaine may therefore sometimes relieve asthma. In the second place the centre for bronchial constriction may be depressed, e.g. by hypnotics or even general anaesthetics. Both these methods are, however, not devoid of danger. Some cases of cocaine addiction have resulted from its use by asthmatics. A safer and more generally applicable method is to give a drug which acts peripherally on the muscle, and there are three ways in which this can be done. The vagal (motor) fibres can be depressed or paralysed by *Atropine* (p. 160) or *Hyoscine* (p. 163). The muscle itself can be relaxed by a direct action, e.g. by nitrites (p. 184). Lastly, the 'terminations' of the sympathetic (dilator) nerve can be 'stimulated', e.g. by *Adrenaline* (p. 169), *Isoprenaline* (p. 172), or *Ephedrine* (p. 172). Sympathetic stimulation is generally the most suitable; it does not dry up the bronchial secretion, which is often a disadvantage with vagal paralysis. *Injection of Adrenaline*, B.P., *Epinephrine Injection*, U.S.P., is widely used for the relief of asthmatic attacks. It is given hypodermically. Small doses, e.g. (3 min.), sometimes suffice at first, but they may have to be increased. Relief is often immediate, but adrenaline has no effect on the cause of asthma and is therefore only indirectly, if at all, curative. *Isoprenaline Sulphate*, B.P., *Isoproterenol Hydrochloride*, U.S.P., is more potent than adrenaline in relaxing the bronchi. It may be administered as a spray or aerosol for inhalation or as a tablet sublingually.

Ephedrine, though often less certain and less prompt in action than adrenaline, has the great merit that it can produce its effects when given by mouth—an especial advantage in the case of children. Also its effect is more prolonged than that of adrenaline.

These sympathomimetic compounds are cardiac stimulants and may give rise to uncomfortable palpitations. Ephedrine is apt to cause wakefulness and sometimes retention of urine especially in older male patients.

XVII

DRUGS WHICH INFLUENCE METABOLISM, BLOOD, ETC.

IODIDES

SEEING that in two important therapeutic uses—in thyroid diseases and in syphilis—the action of iodides can fairly be described as an action on metabolism, iodides can perhaps most conveniently be taken here.

The salt most commonly used medicinally is iodide of potassium, but the actions to be described occur equally well with sodium iodide or indeed with any compound which will liberate the iodide ion. Iodine itself is used chiefly as an antiseptic (p. 250); it is more irritating to the stomach than iodides, so that the latter are usually preferred for oral administration, the actions of iodine and iodides after absorption being identical.

Potassium iodide forms colourless crystals which have a pungent and somewhat bitter salt taste and are freely soluble in water. Large doses, especially if concentrated, irritate the stomach and may produce nausea and vomiting, but this rarely occurs from medicinal use. Iodides are absorbed very rapidly from the alimentary canal and, in their subsequent distribution and excretion, generally resemble chlorides and bromides. Of a single dose, therefore, the greater part is rapidly excreted, chiefly in the urine, but also in other secretions such as saliva and milk; while a diminishing part may be retained in the body for some days. A slight diuretic effect may occur from salt action (p. 25), but iodides do not seem to have any specific action on the kidneys.

People vary very much in their sensitiveness to potassium iodide, so much so that it is impossible to describe certain effects as regularly occurring after certain doses. It was found that when repeated doses of iodides were given, certain disagreeable symptoms might appear to which collectively the name *Iodism* was given. Occasionally this may occur after a single dose, and in any case the amount of iodide which can be given before symptoms of iodism appear varies widely in different individuals. The commonest symptoms of iodism are swelling and catarrh of the mucous membrane of the respiratory tract, usually accompanied by a profuse watery secretion. This is shown by swelling of the mucous membrane of the nose, with sneezing and increased secretion. There may be also conjunctivitis, and catarrh of the frontal sinuses with headache. Less commonly, laryngitis, tracheitis, or bronchitis may occur. Various kinds of skin eruptions may also appear, most frequently of an erythematous or papular type. These effects are probably connected with the excretion of iodides by the various surfaces involved.

While these symptoms are to be avoided as far as possible, iodides are frequently administered to produce a minor degree of one of the symptoms, namely, an increased secretion from the trachea and bronchi. In cases of bronchitis, where it is desirable to increase the quantity and diminish the viscidity of the bronchial secretion, potassium iodide is a reliable and valuable expectorant.

Perhaps the most important therapeutic use of potassium iodide is, however, in the treatment of syphilis. It is of value only in the later stages of this disease, especially when ulcers or gummata are present. The fact that it has no remedial effect in early syphilis renders it improbable that it can act by killing the spirochaete. Indeed, everything goes to show that it does not act like mercury, bismuth, or arsenic as a parasiticide. It acts on tissues, in some way not understood, dissolving and removing gummatous tumours. Iodides are also useful in actinomycosis, and sometimes in chronic rheumatism.

Potassium Iodide, B.P., U.S.P., or *Sodium Iodide*, B.P., U.S.P., are given in doses of 0·3 G. (5 gr.) or less as expectorants, and 0·3–2 G. (5–30 gr.) in the treatment of tertiary syphilis. In actinomycosis much larger doses are often given.

Iodine is an essential constituent of thyroid **hormone and** iodides have important uses in the prophylaxis and treatment of thyroid diseases. To save repetition, these uses can be more conveniently considered along with thyroid (p. 212).

COLCHICINE

Preparations made from the corm or seeds of *Colchicum autumnale*, a plant which grows in meadows and pastures over large areas of Europe and N. Africa, have been used since the Middle Ages as a remedy for gout. The chief active principle of the plant is an alkaloid *Colchicine*, B.P., U.S.P., 0·5 mg. ($\frac{1}{120}$ gr.).

Colchicine is an intense local irritant. It is excreted by the intestines and by the kidney and, when given in large doses, produces an inflammatory irritation of these organs, with resultant nausea, vomiting, and diarrhoea, and sometimes anuria. Medicinal doses ought not to produce effects other than nausea or slight purging. Colchicum also has an action like pilocarpine on smooth muscle, and causes an increased leucocytosis after a temporary leucopenia. It has a curious effect on dividing cells, preventing the completion of mitosis.

None of its actions can at the present time explain its beneficial action in gout. In acute cases of this disease it relieves the pain in the joints, but seems to have little effect in preventing subsequent attacks. It may be given in the form of *Tincture of Colchicum*, B.P., 0·3–1 ml. (5–15 min.).

Cinchophen, B.P., or phenylquinoline carboxylic acid, has a remarkable effect on the kidney in rendering it permeable to uric acid. It increases the amount of uric acid in the urine while causing temporarily a corresponding fall in the concentration in the blood. This increased excretion of uric acid seems to improve some cases of gout, in which disease urates are unduly retained. Like many aromatic substances, cinchophen has also an antipyretic and analgesic action. In gout it may be given in doses of 1·8 G. (30 gr.) a day, in divided doses, on two consecutive days and repeated after a week. It should be given only under close supervision as severe and even fatal hepatitis has occurred from its use. Salicylates also increase the excretion of uric acid and are less toxic.

COAGULATION OF THE BLOOD

The functional value of having the blood endowed with the potentiality of clotting lies in the natural arrest of haemorrhage when a blood vessel is torn or severed. What happens if this mechanism fails to function is seen in a 'bleeding disease', haemophilia, in which rupture of a small blood vessel may lead to severe haemorrhage. But it is equally important that the blood should not clot inside the vessels, as that would stop the circulation through the region supplied by the blocked vessel, as actually occurs in some pathological conditions that give rise to intravascular clotting. The method of coagulation is an ingenious mechanism to provide for the first eventuality and to prevent the second.

The end-point of coagulation is the conversion of a soluble protein, *fibrinogen*, which exists in the blood plasma, into an insoluble, stringy, adherent protein, *fibrin*. This is brought about by the action of an enzyme, *thrombin*, which does not exist in the circulating blood and for the formation of which at least three main factors are necessary: (1) *prothrombin*, (2) *ionized calcium*, both of which exist in the blood, and (3) an enzyme, *thrombokinase* or *thromboplastin*, which does not exist in the plasma but is liberated from injured blood platelets or tissues when blood is shed or there is local trauma. All the factors necessary for coagulation—fibrinogen, prothrombin, and soluble calcium salts—are therefore present in the circulating blood, with the exception of thrombokinase. This absence of thrombokinase normally prevents intravascular clotting together with the presence of fibrinolysin, an enzyme which reverses the coagulation of fibrinogen; on the other hand, all the ingredients are ready in the blood for extra-vascular clotting, provided that the thrombokinase is forthcoming.

We can only briefly consider here (1) remedies which can be used to favour extravascular clotting, should that fail to take place (coagulants), and (2) remedies which prevent intravascular clotting, if that tendency should exist (anticoagulants).

COAGULANTS. Defect of coagulation is very rarely due to lack either of fibrinogen or of ionized calcium in the plasma. Lack of prothrombin occurs in Vitamin K deficiency and can be counteracted by giving Vitamin K or *Menaphthone*, B.P., U.S.P. (p. 238). Lack of a co-factor called antihaemophilic globulin, which controls utilization of thromboplastin, occurs in haemophilia, a congenital disease characterized by delay in the coagulation-time of the blood and by a tendency to recurrent haemorrhages, often from trivial injuries. No very satisfactory treatment of this disease is yet available. Transfusion of whole blood may be the most reliable expedient when the haemorrhage is inaccessible.

For local application various agents may be tried. One of the most powerful coagulants is Russell's viper venom, which has to be used with circumspection. Tannic acid and perchloride of iron favour clotting (but not very efficiently) by coagulating blood proteins. Adrenaline will diminish bleeding by constriction of the arterioles and venules, so facilitating clotting.

Oxidized Cellulose, U.S.P., is an absorbable gauze or cotton which forms an artificial clot when applied to bleeding surfaces. The substance does not enter into the normal clotting mechanism but cellulosic acid has a powerful affinity for haemoglobin.

Absorbable Gelatin Sponge, U.S.P., is insoluble but slowly digested and absorbed from the site of implantation. It should be moistened with saline before application to oozing surfaces.

Thrombin, U.S.P., is used as a powder or in solution for topical application. It must never be injected. It is the natural clotting factor formed by adding thrombokinase preparations to bovine prothrombin with added calcium. It will clot blood, plasma, or fibrinogen in solution.

ANTICOAGULANTS. Intravascular clotting (thrombosis) may occur in certain diseases, e.g. arteriosclerosis, diabetes, typhoid fever, and pneumonia; or may result from conditions which favour stagnation of the blood flow, e.g. in enforced immobility after operations, fractures, &c. Thrombosis often begins in a vein of the leg muscles and may extend indefinitely; or a portion of the clot may separate off and be carried through the right side of the heart to form a pulmonary embolism, which may cause sudden death if the embolus is large. The prophylaxis or treatment of intravascular clotting is, therefore, important.

Heparin, B.P., *Heparin Sodium*, U.S.P., is a substance first obtained from mammalian liver (whence its name) but now usually made from the lungs or other tissues of animals used by man for food. Structurally it is the sodium salt of a complex organic acid containing chondroitin combined with sulphuric acid. It inhibits the activation of prothrombin into thrombin by virtue of its possessing a strongly electro-negative charge. It requires biological assay and the usual dose is 6,000–10,000 Units by intramuscular or intravenous injection, for which there is an *Injection of Heparin*, B.P., *Heparin Sodium Injection*, U.S.P. Since heparin acts on clotting substances present in circulating blood, its action is rapid but of short duration. It usually has to be given four or five times a day by intravenous injection, but more efficiently as a slow intravenous drip of 6,000–12,000 Units in 1 litre of saline solution at such a rate as to maintain the blood clotting time at 15 minutes. Cumulative effects are the more easily avoided as normal coagulability is soon restored when administration is stopped. If haemorrhages occur due to overdosage they can readily be checked by an intravenous injection of Protamine Sulphate. This is an electro-positive polypeptide.

DICOUMAROL

A liability to haemorrhages in cattle was traced to their eating improperly cured clover, and the substance in clover responsible for this, dicoumarol, was isolated, has been synthesized, and is now used for the prophylaxis and treatment of intravascular clotting. It can be used as an alternative or as an adjunct to heparin.

Dicoumarol delays the formation of prothrombin in the liver, possibly by preventing the liver cells from utilizing Vitamin K in the normal continuous synthesis of prothrombin. It acts, therefore, in the opposite direction to Vitamin K (p. 238), by which, in fact, its effects may be counteracted. It is slower in action (1–3 days) than heparin, from which it differs also in having no action on blood *in vitro*. It is effective given by mouth (50–300 mg.), but is absorbed slowly and somewhat erratically. There is also a delay while it exerts its effect by the indirect mechanism described, and as excretion is slow it tends, if treatment is prolonged, to accumulate to a dangerous degree, in which case bleeding may occur. Haematuria is the commonest first sign of this complication. It is therefore necessary to control the action, not by measuring blood clotting time but by measuring blood prothrombin levels. Dicoumarol is not now official in the B.P. but the U.S.P. has a similar compound, **Bishydroxycoumarin**. The action of dicoumarol is delayed, persistent, and difficult to control. Newer, related compounds have been introduced with improved properties.

Ethyl Biscoumacetate, B.P., has replaced dicoumarol because of its much greater speed of effectiveness (18 hours) and the shortness of its action (3 days), which makes it easier to control the delicate balance between haemorrhage and thrombus. The dose is 0·15–1 G. per day, given until prothrombin time is reduced to about 30 seconds.

Phenindione, B.P., initial dose 0·2–0·3 G., is equally speedy and effective, but lasts for 24 hours only. Structurally it is not a coumarin derivative.

THERAPEUTIC USES. Anticoagulants are used to prevent the extension of established clot as, for example, in coronary thrombosis and in venous thrombosis of the limbs, and to help in the lysis of the thrombus rather than its organization. Heparin gives the most rapid effect but coumarin derivatives are much easier to administer and exert much more prolonged effects, thus being useful to keep the blood from undesirable clotting in auricular fibrillation or after vascular surgery.

XVIII

HORMONES

The numerous glands of the body can be divided into two groups—glands of external secretion and glands of internal secretion. The former discharge their secretions outside the body proper, e.g. lachrymal, salivary, gastro-intestinal, bronchial, and sweat glands; the latter discharge their secretions into the blood.

Generally speaking, glands of the former group perform functions which must be called into effect quickly but which are of relatively transient duration, e.g. minutes or hours. This timing of action largely holds good also for all kinds of muscle. This type of prompt, transient action is concerned mainly with two functions: (*a*) movement of some kind, and (*b*) immediate glandular responses to changes in environment. Of the latter influences the most important are: (1) the entrance of food into the alimentary canal (salivary and gastro-intestinal glands), (2) the entrance of air into the lungs (bronchial glands), and (3) changes in external temperature (sweat glands). Such actions are in the main under control of the nervous system, though even here mediated by chemical transmitters (Chap. XII).

On the other hand there are many other requirements of the body, notably the growth of the skeleton and of the reproductive organs and the slower kinds of metabolic changes, which may require longer time for their fulfilment days or even years, and for which speed of action is relatively less urgent. For these a milder and more enduring form of stimulus is more appropriate and these effects are now known to be largely controlled by hormones, chemical substances secreted by the second group of glands—those of internal secretion.

Advances in physiological and chemical knowledge are steadily bringing to light more and more hormones and emphasizing the important part they play in the animal economy. Any complete consideration of them would involve a large part of physiology. It will be possible here to consider only those hormones which, either in the form of extracts of the glands concerned or in the form of their active principles, are available for therapeutic use and which have attained a reasonably assured place in the treatment of disease.

THYROID GLAND

The internal secretion of the thyroid gland is essential for normal development and health, as is shown by the remarkable effects resulting from *deficiency* of it. Congenital deficiency (*cretinism*) arrests and warps development, affecting probably all organs more or less, but conspicuously the skeletal structures, the integument, the nervous system, and metabolism. The child is dwarfed, with thick dry skin, coarse hair, and protuberant abdomen. Mental and sexual development is retarded and the basal metabolism is low.

In deficiency of thyroid secretion (*myxoedema*), either from pathological causes or as the result of operative removal of the thyroid gland, the effects are very similar, except that, in adults, growth has been complete before the deficiency comes on.

In such conditions, more or less complete recovery may result from thyroid administration. In cretinism the earlier the treatment is begun the better are the results, and administration of thyroid must be continued during life. The exact dose necessary to maintain normal metabolism must be determined for each case. Thyroid administration is also useful in less severe forms of thyroid deficiency. The decrease in weight and rise in basal metabolism resulting from thyroid medication have suggested its use in obesity, which it sometimes temporarily reduces. Overdosage with thyroid produces symptoms similar to those seen in exophthalmic goitre (p. 214).

Thyroid Deficiencies

Thyroid deficiencies (cretinism or myxoedema) may be treated by giving **Thyroid**, B.P., U.S.P., a cream-coloured amorphous powder, prepared from the thyroid glands of oxen, sheep, or pigs; dose: B.P., 30–240 mg. ($\frac{1}{2}$–4 gr.) daily; U.S.P., 60 mg.: conveniently given in the form of tablets. The B.P. preparation contains 0·1 per cent. (U.S.P. 0·2 per cent.) of iodine in combination as thyroxine.

In the gland iodine combines with amino-acid to form diiodo-tyrosine which is further modified to tetraiodothyronine or thyroxine, the structure of which is shown below. It is stored in the colloid of the gland as the protein thyroglobulin. The form in which the hormone is secreted into the blood is not finally determined, but it may be as triiodothyronine (formed by re-moval of one I from thyroxine) which has been found in the blood and which is more active than thyroxine. Thyroid takes about 7–10 days to exert its full effect.

$$\text{HO} \diagdown \!\!\! \diagup \text{O} \diagdown \!\!\! \diagup CH_2 \cdot CH \cdot NH_2 \cdot COOH. \qquad \text{Thyroxine.}$$

Thyroxine Sodium, which forms white crystalline needles, insoluble in water but soluble in strong alkalis may be pre-ferred to thyroid. It takes 3–4 days to exert a maximum effect, given in doses of 0·1 mg. increased gradually as needed.

Treatment of Simple Goitre

A goitre is a swelling in the neck due to enlargement of the thyroid gland.

The thyroid gland contains a much higher content of iodine than the other tissues of the body, and the iodine necessary for the continual manufacture of thyroxin is obtained from the food, which only exceptionally fails to furnish the very small amount necessary. This may occur, however, especially in dis-tricts remote from the sea, where the drinking water is deficient in iodine. There goitre may be endemic. The very variable degree of enlargement is due to distension of the acini or to adenomatous cysts and is not usually accompanied by exces-sive secretion of thyroid hormone. Iodides here prove very successful in the *prophylaxis* of endemic simple goitre; they may be administered by adding minute amounts of iodide to common salt or by giving for ten days, in spring and autumn, about 0·2 G. (3 gr.) daily. Iodides are less effective in the *treatment* of established simple goitre, but may relieve it. If the enlargement is too unsightly or causes pressure symptoms or if symptoms of hyperthyroidism arise, surgical treatment may be necessary.

Treatment of Toxic Goitre

In this condition there is a hyperplasia of the thyroid gland leading to an excessive secretion of thyroid hormone. Among the numerous symptoms are goitre (not always proportional to the severity of the symptoms); tachycardia, often leading to auricular fibrillation; exophthalmos (protuberant eyeballs); increased metabolism with loss of weight; fine tremor, especially of the muscles of the fingers, and weakness of the voluntary muscles.

In severe hyperthyroidism the prognosis was formerly very grave, many cases dying from progressive heart-failure with auricular fibrillation or from other thyrotoxic symptoms. The condition could be improved by operative removal of part of the thyroid gland, but the mortality from operation was high. The outlook was entirely changed by the discovery of the value of pre-operative administration of iodine or iodides. When these are given (small doses, e.g. 60 mg. (1 gr.) of potassium iodide twice daily, are sufficient), a marked suppression of the thyrotoxic symptoms is usually produced, reaching an optimum in about 10–14 days. The operation has to be timed to coincide with this period. As a result of this pre-operative treatment, and with improvements in operative and anaesthetic technique, the mortality from thyroidectomy has been greatly reduced, and the prognosis for complete subsequent recovery is now good.

RADIOACTIVE IODINE. As iodine is specifically concentrated in the thyroid gland, it is possible by giving radioactive iodine to deliver a high local dose of radiation to functioning thyroid tissue, with a minimum effect on other organs, as the beta radiation emitted by the isotope scarcely travels beyond the capsule of the gland. Thyrotoxicosis can often be controlled by radioactive iodine, which is also of value in some cases of thyroid carcinoma. *Sodium Radio-Iodide I^131 Solution*, U.S.P., is specially prepared for this form of administration.

THIOURACILS

In 1943 a new method of treating hyperthyroidism was introduced by the discovery that thiouracil, a thiopyrimidine compound, could produce a marked relief of thyrotoxic symptoms; e.g. fall in metabolic rate, increase of weight, cessation of flushing, sometimes even stoppage of auricular fibrillation, as well as a pronounced subjective improvement. Thiouracil seems to act by interfering with the synthesis of thyroxin, probably by preventing the iodization of tyrosine. It has now been widely used for the relief of thyrotoxicosis, improvement beginning in a week and reaching a maximum in two or three months. Care must be taken to find a maintenance dose just sufficient to ensure thyroid equilibrium. This method of treatment may produce complete suppression of the symptoms of hyperthyroidism, but not regression of the exophthalmos or the goitre.

Methylthiouracil, B.P., controlling dose 0·2–0·6 G. daily, maintenance dose 50–200 mg. daily, U.S.P., 200 mg. daily; acts similarly and as it produces less side effects has now replaced thiouracil.

Propylthiouracil, B.P., U.S.P., in the same dosage is more active and safer and usually preferred. To prepare for operative interference it is given in doses of 0·1 G. 8-hourly and is more effective than the earlier treatment with iodine or iodide. Among the toxic symptoms that may occur with thiouracils are fever, skin rashes, oedema of the face or ankles. The most serious is agranulocytosis (p. 127). Treatment should be controlled by blood counts.

Methimazole, U.S.P., is again more potent, quicker acting and perhaps less toxic. The dosage is 10 mg. every 8 hours until control is effected, a matter of 1–2 months. The maintenance dose has to be found by trial and error.

PARATHYROID GLAND

Complete removal of the parathyroid glands causes death in a few days owing to lack of a hormone necessary to life, which these glands secrete into the blood. Among the effects resulting from removal of the parathyroids is a lowering of the blood-calcium, with a consequent increase in muscular irritability giving rise to tetany. An extract of the gland can be prepared which contains this hormone, and which, when injected, causes a rapid rise in the serum calcium and relieves tetany if present. Parathyroid extract increases the blood-calcium by withdrawing calcium from the bones or soft tissues, not by increasing its absorption. It produces therefore only a temporary effect. It has been used tentatively in a number of pathological conditions, but especially in tetany. *Parathyroid Injection*, U.S.P., average dose 50 U.S.P. Units daily by injection.

Tumour of the parathyroid, leading to prolonged excessive secretion of the hormone, may produce osteitis fibrosa, the bones being easily broken owing to decalcification.

THE PANCREAS: INSULIN

Insulin is a preparation made from the pancreas and containing the active hormone of the islets (*insulae*) of the gland, whence its name. It was shown, many years ago, that removal of the pancreas in animals produced symptoms similar to those of diabetes mellitus in man; and, about fifty years ago, that these symptoms could be prevented by pancreatic grafts. It was not until 1922, however, that Banting and Best were successful in obtaining from the pancreas an active preparation containing the hormone in a state of sufficient purity to be used in diabetic patients. To this preparation they gave the name insulin.

Insulin, a protein, destroyed by pepsin and trypsin, has no action when given by mouth. When injected subcutaneously, it causes a fall in blood-sugar, the degree of fall depending upon the dose administered. The effect is produced in normal animals and, with smaller doses, in diabetic patients, and is due to the fact that insulin increases the capacity of the tissues to take up and metabolize sugar. In diabetes mellitus this capacity is partly or wholly lost, due to lack of the normal internal secretion of the islets of Langerhans. Administration of insulin supplies this defect, and must be regulated according to the severity of the diabetes. Insulin therapy of diabetes, therefore, is analogous to thyroid treatment of myxoedema. It is not a permanent cure, and, unless the pancreas recovers its normal power of secreting the hormone, insulin must be given more or less continuously, as may be necessary.

Although the exact chemical composition of insulin is known, the activity of it is determined physiologically in terms of units per ml., the preparation to be tested being compared with a standard preparation. The criterion of comparative activity used may be the percentage fall of blood sugar produced in rabbits or the symptoms of hypoglycaemia produced in mice. One mg. of the standard preparation contains 22 Units of activity. In diabetes daily doses of 5–40 Units or more may be given, depending upon the severity of the disease and the amount of carbohydrate allowed in the diet. *Injection of Insulin*, B.P., *Insulin Injection*, U.S.P., is official in several strengths each with a distinctive coloured label. The usual strength is 40 Units per ml.

In diabetes the sugar in the blood is increased mainly because of diminished utilization together with decreased storage of glycogen in the liver. There is an associated increase in fat metabolism, often with the formation of ketone bodies such as aceto-acetic acid which may produce exaggerated respiration (air hunger), or coma. This diabetic coma is usually treated by giving insulin and sugar together, so as to decrease the formation of ketone bodies.

In a healthy person the normal secretion of insulin by the pancreas is so regulated as to maintain a fairly constant level of blood-sugar. On the other hand, a single injection of insulin in a diabetic, if effective, tends to produce too great and too transient a fall in blood sugar. Various methods have been tried to obtain a degree and rate of absorption of insulin corresponding more closely to its normal secretion and to avoid the necessity of frequent injections and the risk of accidental hypoglycaemia. This is done by combining with insulin substances which delay its action. The following preparations are official and are additional to the simple Injection of Insulin already mentioned.

Insulin Zinc Suspension, B.P., is a sterile buffered suspension of insulin with zinc chloride, available in the B.P. in three physical forms: *Insulin Zinc Suspension (Amorphous), Insulin Zinc Suspension (Crystalline)* and *Insulin Zinc Suspension,* which is a mixture of three volumes of the Amorphous with seven volumes of the Crystalline Suspension.

Injection of Protamine Zinc Insulin, B.P., *Protamine Zinc Insulin Injection,* U.S.P., is amorphous in structure, as is *Isophane Insulin Injection,* U.S.P. They are prepared by mixing appropriate amounts of insulin, fish sperm protamine, zinc chloride, and glycerin together, and adding a buffered solution to the suspension. *Injection of Globin Zinc Insulin,* B.P., *Globin Zinc Insulin Injection,* U.S.P., is produced by adding appropriate amounts of globin, zinc chloride, and glycerin to insulin. It must be clearly realized that these and other available insulins are only forms of the one active hormone and that the purpose behind them is the attempt to imitate the natural time-intervals of release of the islet secretion. They vary in the speed of onset, time of peak activity and total intensity, and duration of their action as follows. Onset: Unmodified Insulin 1 hr., Globin Insulin 1–2 hrs., Insulin Zinc Suspension 2 hrs., Protamine Zinc Insulin 4–6 hrs.; time of peak action (in the same order): 2–3 hrs., 6–12 hrs., 10–20 hrs., and 16–24 hrs.; duration of action: 6–8 hrs., 18–24 hrs., 20–30 hrs., 24–36 hrs. or longer. Adjustments must be made in the regimen of the patient in timing injections and food consumption to avoid over- or underactivity.

If too much insulin is given, symptoms of *hypoglycaemia* occur. The normal amount of glucose in the blood is about 100 mg. per 100 ml. If the blood sugar is reduced to below two-thirds of this amount, symptoms such as sweating, faintness, tremulousness, and a feeling of anxiety may come on. If the sugar is reduced to 50 mg. per 100 ml., aphasia, delirium, convulsions, or even coma and death may ensue. Diabetics vary considerably in regard to the toxic symptoms induced by a given degree of hypoglycaemia. Symptoms of hypoglycaemia can be rapidly relieved by the administration of sugar by mouth or, if necessary, by vein; or adrenaline can be used in emergency, as it causes hyperglycaemia. Use has been made of this hypoglycaemic convulsive reaction in the treatment of severe psychotic disorders.

Given in correct dosage, insulin causes a remarkable alleviation of the symptoms of diabetes. Accompanying the fall in the sugar of the blood there is diminished glycosuria, polyuria, and thirst; and, with the aid of insulin and suitable diet, many diabetics can continue active physical and mental work. As the dosage requirements vary so much in different patients, no official doses are given for insulin preparations. It is merely recommended that doses must be determined according to the needs of the patient.

ADRENAL CORTEX

Cholesterol occurs in all animal cells, and substances possessing its basic carbon skeleton are called sterols. They differ in the type and arrangement of attached groups which make a large number of compounds possible, with differences in their physiological activity. Some of these sterols, derived from cholesterol, form a group of related compounds of fundamental importance in regulating various functions of the body. Among these are the steroids secreted by the adrenal cortex.

Cortisone.

The adrenal cortex is necessary to life. Removal causes an

abnormal loss of sodium chloride from the body with coincident loss of water and a retention of potassium. Blood volume is reduced, blood pressure falls, low blood-sugar levels and high nitrogen levels occur; there is progressive muscular weakness and death may follow. Similar symptoms are found in Addison's disease and more acutely in the Friderichsen–Waterhouse syndrome, which are due to pathological involvement of the gland. Relief from these symptoms and prolongation of life can be produced by administration of active extracts of adrenal cortex along with liberal administration of sodium chloride and restriction of potassium. Cortical extracts have to be injected parenterally and potency is very variable; they have been replaced by purified crystalline corticosteroids. The cortical steroids are usually classified as: (1) mineralo-corticoids which control mineral and water metabolism, e.g. *Deoxycortone*; (2) glucocorticoids which influence carbohydrate and protein metabolism, e.g. *Cortisone* and *Hydrocortisone*, and (3) sex hormones, e.g. *Progesterone*, an androgen and an oestrogen. This classification is unsatisfactory in that all these effects overlap to a greater or lesser degree in the different compounds. The function of these substances in combination is to maintain a state of balance in the internal environment of an organism in the face of a changing environment. They are produced by synthesis from cholesterol and liberated as a result of ACTH activity (p. 224), by discharge of adrenal medullary hormone (adrenaline, noradrenaline) in states of activity, or by changes in blood Na/K ratio, among other things. When injected they disappear rapidly and are ultimately excreted in the urine in the form of 17-ketosteroids.

The mode of action of these substances is still obscure and here it is possible only to give a brief description of the complicated actions and bewildering range of therapeutic uses of those compounds which are at present widely used.

Deoxycortone Acetate, B.P., *Desoxycorticosterone Acetate*, U.S.P., (Deoxycortone) was synthesized in 1937 and the acetate (DOCA) was soon commercially available and found to be very effective in the treatment of Addison's disease. Especially it restored the mineral and water metabolism, the aberrations of which in this disease have been mentioned above. Though patients with adrenal deficiencies could be kept alive with adequate doses of deoxycortone, it did not provide complete replacement. Patients remained liable to hypoglycaemic attacks and a severe stress might precipitate a dangerous crisis. Nevertheless it was an important therapeutic advance. Especially milder cases of Addison's disease could be successfully treated by giving large amounts of sodium and restricting potassium, supplemented by deoxycortone. If this failed in acute crises of the disease, extract of the adrenal cortex could be used. The main use of deoxycortone is therefore to control mineral metabolism in cases of adrenal deficiency. The acetate is given parenterally, B.P. 2–5 mg. daily, for which there is an official intramuscular *Injection*. A slower and more prolonged absorption (which avoids frequent injections) can be obtained by the use of an *Implant*, B.P. (0·1–0·4 G.), or *Pellet*, U.S.P., which is inserted subcutaneously to form a depot from which gradual absorption takes place.

Cortisone. Cortisone was synthesized in 1946 and was found to have a wider range of action than deoxycortone.

1. It has important effects on carbohydrate and protein metabolism. Gluconeogenesis from protein is stimulated, leading to increased storage of glycogen in the liver. There may be a rise in blood-sugar with glycosuria and the sensitivity to insulin is decreased. By increasing conversion of protein to carbohydrate, large doses induce a negative nitrogen balance with an increased secretion of uric acid.

2. Large doses cause increased sodium retention with increased potassium loss. Overdosage may cause excessive sodium retention with consequent oedema due to water retention.

Both these actions counteract the salient effects of adrenal deficiency. Factor (1) supplements the action on carbohydrate metabolism which, as has been mentioned, is lacking with deoxycortone. Severe cases of Addison's disease were therefore more adequately treated by a combination of both steroids, which came nearer to possessing the active steroids found in an extract of the cortex. Actually some authorities now believe that, with judicious dosage, Addison's disease can be successfully treated by cortisone alone.

3. Cortisone was found to have other remarkable effects, which have given it a wide range of therapeutic uses, other than in gross adrenal deficiency, of which the following may be mentioned.

It is believed to improve the body's response to stress, though this is perhaps a somewhat vague claim. Factually it affects inflammatory reactions by diminishing capillary permeability, inhibiting the formation of granulation tissue and the fibroblastic reaction of repair. This it does regardless of the type of infection. It may thus suppress a detrimental fever and toxaemia accompanying inflammation, but at the risk of interfering with the normal protective reaction of inflammation. It does not kill infective agents or *cure* diseases due to them.

It has a dramatic effect in many allergic diseases in some of which it may be life-saving. These include urticaria, hay-fever, angioneurotic oedema, exfoliative dermatitis and drug allergies. It is specially valuable in resistant cases of status asthmaticus and in many more chronic diseases such as polyarteritis, disseminated lupus, pemphigus, ulcerative colitis, hypopituitarism, leukaemia, rheumatoid arthritis. Among toxic effects which may occur are 'moonface', sodium retention, disturbance of sex hormone balance, breakdown of old tubercular foci, delayed healing of fractures, exacerbation of peptic ulcer or of diabetes.

Cortisone Acetate, B.P., U.S.P., 12·5–50 mg. daily as a maintenance dose for replacement therapy; 50–100 mg. to control inflammatory processes; 200–400 mg. in some acute emergencies. In general it is best given by mouth, e.g. as a tablet, but exceptionally it may be given by intramuscular injection.

Hydrocortisone was synthesized in 1950. It acts qualitatively like cortisone but is more soluble and more potent in the treatment of some inflammatory diseases. It may be given by mouth or as an injection, dosage being about two-thirds that of cortisone. It has a great advantage in that it is very effective by local application, and *Hydrocortisone Acetate*, U.S.P., is used in an ointment for skin conditions, especially pruritus ani and vulvae and in infantile eczema. It relieves itching, and oedema and erythema are suppressed. A very important use is in inflammatory conditions of the eye, especially in acute iritis and iridocyclitis, when it blocks the inflammatory phase and may prevent cataract or glaucoma. It is given as eye-drops and no systemic effects are produced.

Aldosterone is a more recent addition to the corticosteroids. It is closely related chemically to cortisone and deoxycortone but differs in containing an aldehyde group, whence its name. It is more potent than deoxycortone in controlling electrolyte metabolism and appears to have also some effect on carbohydrate metabolism. It has not yet been available in sufficient quantity to establish its particular therapeutic value.

Prednisone and *Prednisolone* are derivatives of cortisone and hydrocortisone respectively. Prednisone acetate is fully effective, given by mouth or by injection, in smaller amounts than cortisone itself. The main advantage claimed for it is that it is effective in rheumatoid arthritis and in other collagen diseases, and in allergic states and skin diseases, while having only slight effect on electrolyte metabolism, so that sodium retention is not likely to interfere with its therapeutic use.

PITUITARY GLAND (ANTERIOR LOBE)

The pituitary is a *multum in parvo* gland which secretes a number of important hormones. The hormones of the posterior lobe have their most important actions on involuntary muscle (p. 178) and on the kidney (p. 24) and are therefore more conveniently discussed elsewhere.

The functions of the anterior lobe fall to be considered here. The hormones secreted by it are of two kinds: (1) a hormone which produces its effects by a direct action on tissues, and (2) hormones which act mainly by stimulating other glands to secrete their particular hormones; they are so to speak hormones of hormones.

(1) The most conspicuous action of the growth hormone

is to control the growth of the skeleton. When an eosinophil adenoma of the gland, which causes excessive secretion of this hormone, develops in a patient before the epiphyses have fused there is a generalized overgrowth of the skeleton, producing *gigantism*. If the tumour occurs in an adult it produces *acromegaly*, with overgrowth of the bones, noticeably of the face and of the hands and feet. Pressure symptoms due to tumour, disturbances of metabolism and of sexual function are common.

Deficiency of this hormone causes a symmetrical retardation of skeletal growth, 'dwarfism', with usually no mental impairment, such as is seen in cretinism.

(2) From extracts of the anterior lobe several protein hormones can be separated, differing from one another and having the functions of stimulating other endocrine glands to secrete their individual hormones. Glands so influenced include the adrenal cortex, thyroid, and sex glands. Removal of the pituitary causes atrophy of these glands, injection of pituitary extracts overactivity of them. Mutual reactions of the pituitary and of these glands serve to maintain an optimum balance of various of these hormones in the blood. It will be possible here to consider only those which have been separated so as to be used as therapeutic agents.

Corticotrophin, B.P., (Adrenocorticotrophic Hormone) is a polypeptide extracted from the anterior pituitary of pigs, which is partially purified and biologically assayed. To take the name piecemeal in reverse it means the hormone which stimulates the cortex of the adrenals. This formidable name, in this age of initials, has commonly been referred to in the literature as ACTH. It is absorbed from parenteral injection but is inactive when given by mouth, *Injection of Corticotrophin*, B.P., *Corticotropin Injection*, U.S.P., 10 Units intravenously, well diluted. It is rather unstable and hence must be administered within one month of preparation. It disappears rapidly from the blood after injection and is thus more effective if well diluted and given by intravenous drip over a period of 6–8 hours.

As has been previously discussed (p. 219), conditions of adrenal deficiency and a variety of other disorders can be effectively treated by administering cortical hormones such as cortisone and hydrocortisone. Corticotrophin on the other hand stimulates the cortex to secrete its own hormones. Its action is to bring about a proliferation of all the cortex with consequent release of greater or less amounts of all the cortical hormones—a blunderbuss method of treatment, as in a particular case some hormones may be unnecessary or even disadvantageous. Among its effects are decreased excretion of sodium, which may produce oedema, rise of blood-sugar levels, reduced carbohydrate tolerance, virilism (hairiness and acne), muscular weakness (potassium depletion), absence of menses (suppression of ovarian activity). Naturally it would be a poor therapeutic agent if given in doses large enough to produce all these effects. The practical problem has been to discover the selective effects of small doses of corticotrophin and whether it is superior therapeutically to the effects of single or combined administration of individual cortical hormones.

Corticotrophin has been found effective in many of the diseases which respond well to cortisone, but not in Addison's disease as the diseased adrenal cannot secrete the steroids, even under stimulus. It has been used especially in allergic states, e.g. asthma, urticaria, angioneurotic oedema, and in rheumatoid arthritis.

Among other hormones secreted by the anterior pituitary are thyrotrophin, which stimulates the thyroid secretion; prolactin, which stimulates milk secretion; and gonadotrophins.

FEMALE SEX HORMONES

The human ovary may be regarded as a gland, but it differs from other glands in that its primary function is not to discharge an active secretion but to liberate a living cell—the ovum. This it does once a month during reproductive life with praiseworthy regularity, in the hope—usually a forlorn hope—that the ovum will be fertilized and grow into a viable foetus. But the ovary is also a true secreting gland, the hormones that it secretes being concerned with changes in the reproductive organs, the nature of which varies according to the fate of the liberated ovum. The objects of these changes are, briefly, as follows: (1) to get the endometrium into a condition adapted for implantation of the fertilized ovum; (2) if the ovum is fertilized, to maintain its development, to provide for the gradual but enormous growth of the uterine muscle so that it can cope with parturition when the time comes, and to induce an active mammary secretion ready for the child at birth; and (3) if the ovum is not fertilized, to repeat the necessary anticipations for the next ovum. Broadly speaking, the ovarian hormones are so 'designed' that the action of a hormone secreted at one stage of the ovary is to prepare the uterus for the next phase. Several hormones are concerned with the functions of the female reproductive organs. That those organs should require an exceptionally complicated hormone control is the less surprising when we reflect that they may have to undergo more frequent, gross and diverse changes than any other organs in the body. We can here only very briefly refer to those available hormones which have proved of practical therapeutic value.

FOLLICULAR (OESTROGENIC) HORMONES

The Graafian follicles, during their development, secrete hormones called 'oestrogenic' because, when injected into immature or ovariectomized animals, they induce changes in the genital tract characteristic of true oestrus. They control the development of secondary sexual characters, and in the human female produce proliferative and vascular (preovulationary) changes in the endometrium. They also promote the duct system of the breasts.

Three oestrogenic substances have been found in the human female, oestradiol, oestrone, and oestriol. They are steroids closely related chemically to the corticosteroids. Oestradiol, the most powerful, is most generally used. Oestradiol may be used as an ester, *Oestradiol Monobenzoate*, B.P., 1–5 mg.; *Estradiol Benzoate*, U.S.P., 1 mg. They are ineffective when given by mouth and are administered by intramuscular injection, with an oily basis, as they are practically insoluble in water.

The chief uses of oestradiol are in primary amenorrhoea, and in dysmenorrhoea when the pain coincides with the onset of menstruation, acting here probably by increasing the vascularization of the uterus. It is also used for the relief of menopausal symptoms.

Ethinyloestradiol, B.P., U.S.P., is a closely related steroid synthetic derivative of oestradiol. It is the most potent oestrogenic substance known, dosage 0·01–0·1 mg. daily, by mouth for relief of menopausal symptoms—hot flushes and weakness.

SYNTHETIC NON-STEROID OESTROGENS. Several artificial compounds have been found to possess a high oestrogenic activity. Of these, the following are official.

Stilboestrol, B.P., 0·1–5 mg. daily, *Diethylstilbestrol*, U.S.P., 0·5 mg.; and *Dienoestrol*, B.P., U.S.P., 0·5–10 mg. daily. The latter is the less potent but has fewer side-effects and may with advantage be substituted. Synthetic preparations, being cheaper and effective by oral administration, have largely replaced the natural oestrogens in medical practice.

Oestrogens have been given in large doses in the treatment of inoperable carcinoma of the prostate gland with relief of symptoms and prolongation of life. They also inhibit mammary secretion and are much used for this purpose in women in whom for any reason breast feeding is considered undesirable.

CORPUS LUTEUM HORMONE: PROGESTERONE

One follicle in each cycle which has reached full development and released an ovum forms a corpus luteum, which elaborates a specific hormone, progesterone. Its main functions are to change the endometrium from the proliferative to the secretory (premenstrual) phase, and to promote nidification of the fertilized ovum and the maintenance of pregnancy. As the name implies, it prepares for pregnancy. If fertilization fails to occur, the endometrium at the end of the secretory phase breaks down and bleeding (menstruation) follows. Progesterone is also found in the placenta and in the adrenal cortex.

Progesterone, B.P., U.S.P., is used chiefly in the treatment of excessive uterine bleeding (which is often due to defective formation of corpus luteum), dysmenorrhoea, when pain occurs before the onset of menstruation, and habitual or threatened abortion. It is conveniently given intramuscularly as the official *Injection of Progesterone*, B.P., 5–20 mg. daily; U.S.P., 25 mg.

Ethisterone, B.P., U.S.P., a related compound, is active when given by mouth; dose: B.P., 25–100 mg. daily; U.S.P., 10 mg. four times a day; usually as tablets.

GONADOTROPHIC HORMONES: GONADOTROPHINS

Oestradiol and progesterone are hormones secreted by the ovary itself, by the follicles and corpus luteum, respectively. They can be substituted medicinally when the ovary fails to secrete them. But a similar result would be attained if some substance could be given which could stimulate the ovary to produce more of its own secretions. Hormones secreted by the anterior pituitary gland (p. 224) normally exert this influence on the ovaries and hence are called 'gonadotrophic' hormones. Active principles, or even potent extracts, are, however, difficult to prepare from this gland and are unstable, so that they are not yet generally available for therapeutic use.

In the fluids of pregnant animals the following two substances formed by the placenta have been found which resemble in action the true gonadotrophic hormones of the anterior pituitary gland.

Serum Gonadotrophin, B.P., is obtained from the serum of pregnant mares during the middle third of their pregnancy. It stimulates the growth of primordial follicles. It is soluble in water and is given by aqueous intramuscular injection (200–1,000 Units). It is used especially in the treatment of amenorrhoea.

Chorionic Gonadotrophin, B.P., (urine gonadotrophin), is obtained from the urine of pregnant women. It is the basis for the Aschheim-Zondek and Xenopus tests for pregnancy. It does not promote formation of corpora lutea but augments the activity of any already working. Its normal function is probably to maintain pregnancy in the early stages by ensuring dominance of progesterone. Dose, 500–1,000 Units twice weekly.

MALE SEX HORMONES: TESTOSTERONE

In so far as hormone control is concerned, the male sex organs follow the same general plan as the female; that is to say, the testicles secrete hormones which influence the genital organs, and the secretion of these hormones is controlled by gonado-trophic hormones secreted by the anterior pituitary gland.

Testosterone is the most important available hormone. Secreted by the testes, it stimulates the growth and development of the male sexual organs and the development of the secondary sex characters. It does not stimulate spermatogenesis.

It is used chiefly in eunuchoidism, whether due to castration or defective development of the testes. The penis becomes larger and the hair and voice assume the adult male characters. Sexual desire and potency are often increased. It has also been used in some gynaecological conditions, but there is a risk of overdosage producing masculinization, especially hirsutism. *Testosterone*, B.P., U.S.P., is used in the form of *Implants* B.P., total dose 0·1–0·6 G.; *Pellets*, U.S.P., 300 mg.: the effects may last for several months. *Testosterone Propionate*, B.P., 5–25 mg. daily, U.S.P., 25 mg. daily, is given intramuscularly.

Methyltestosterone has the advantage that it acts when given by mouth, B.P., 25–50 mg. (5–20 mg. in women); U.S.P., 10 mg. daily. It is more active when given sublingually, U.S.P., 5 mg. up to four times a day. The uses are the same as of testosterone.

XIX

VITAMINS

VITAMINS are substances occurring in various articles of diet and necessary for insuring normal development and maintaining health, but which act in such small quantities that they cannot be regarded merely, if at all, as sources of energy. A number of vitamins have already been recognized by the effects resulting from their absence in foods or from the positive effects occurring when the deficiency is supplied, and their chemical composition has been gradually revealed.

Until the chemical nature of substances having the properties of vitamins was discovered, vitamins have been designated by alphabetical letters, but advance in knowledge has shown that a preparation originally distinguished alphabetically may contain more than one chemical substance and it is of course preferable that, once a vitamin has been isolated and its chemical structure is known, it should be called by its chemical or other specific name. Of the known vitamins, Vitamins A, D, E, and K are soluble in fats.

VITAMIN A

Vitamin A, soluble in fats and oils, generally occurs in association with some animal fats, such as cod-liver oil or butter, but is absent from vegetable oils like olive oil. The original source of this vitamin is a class of pigments, called carotenes, which are widely distributed in plants and form the red pigment in carrots. Carotenes are converted into Vitamin A in the liver where the vitamin is stored.

Deficiency of Vitamin A causes degeneration and keratinization of epithelial cells, especially in mucous membranes of the conjunctiva (leading to xerophthalmia), of the cornea, and of the trachea and bronchi. These changes may predispose to infections of these surfaces. One of the earliest signs of deficiency is loss of visual acuity in dim light, or night-blindness, apparently due to interference with the regeneration of visual purple. Deafness, incoordination of muscular movements, and deformities of the teeth may also occur from lack of Vitamin A.

The most important dietary sources of carotenes and Vitamin A are green vegetables, carrots, milk, butter, egg-yolk, and liver. For supplementary administration the best and cheapest natural source is a good fish-liver oil. For preparations see p. 237.

VITAMIN B

Aneurine Hydrochloride, B.P., *Thiamine Hydrochloride*, U.S.P., (Vitamin B_1), has been isolated and synthesized. It occurs in the germ and pericarp of cereals, in nuts, yeast, liver, &c. Wholemeal bread and unpolished rice are good sources of it in a diet. Aneurine is necessary as a catalyst for the complete oxidation of carbohydrates, an action which may explain some or all of the effects which result from deficiency of it. Severe deficiency leads to beri-beri, characterized by neuritis, oedema, and cardio-vascular symptoms. Minor deficiency may give rise to anorexia and gastro-intestinal disturbances. A usual dose is 5 mg. daily, but much larger doses, up to 50 mg. daily, are required in severe beri-beri. There seems to be no danger from overdosage. It may be given by injection in cases of neuritis.

A preparation of autoclaved yeast (formerly called vitamin B_2) is now known to contain several factors which are sometimes referred to as 'the vitamin B complex'. Of these factors, the following are believed to be of therapeutic value in man and their composition is known.

Nicotinic Acid, B.P., U.S.P., ($C_5H_4N \cdot COOH$), is a substance of relatively simple constitution, which has long been known; but not until 1937, when it was shown to cure pellagra, was it recognized to be of dietetic importance. It is widely distributed in yeast, liver, milk, cheese, eggs, &c. Pellagra occurs among poorly nourished populations, most commonly in those who live mainly on maize. In England it is recognized occasionally and especially in patients in mental hospitals or those suffering from ulcerative colitis. The characteristic symptoms of pellagra are ulcerations of the mouth and tongue, a characteristic dermatitis, and mental symptoms. These rapidly clear up when nicotinic acid is given. It forms part of the enzyme systems concerned with cellular oxidation. A usual prophylactic dose is 15–30 mg. by mouth daily, but up to 250 mg. a day has been given in pellagra. It is toxic in large amounts, causing flushing, burning and itching of the skin, and increased motility of the stomach.

Nicotinamide, B.P., U.S.P. Nicotinic acid is pyridine-carboxylic acid and the amide of the acid has equal therapeutic properties if given in similar doses. It has the advantage of being less likely to cause vasomotor disturbances.

Riboflavine, B.P., U.S.P., (Lactoflavin), was synthesized in 1935 and occurs as an orange-yellow powder, easily destroyed by light, especially when in solution. It is sparingly soluble in water, giving an intense greenish-yellow fluorescence. It is widely distributed in plants and animals, e.g. in yeast, vegetables, milk, eggs, and liver. Symptoms due to riboflavin deficiency in man include fissures at the angles of the mouth, glossitis, dermatitis, and keratitis. These symptoms are most often seen in such deficiency diseases as pellagra and sprue. Doses, prophylactic 1–4 mg. per day, therapeutic, 5–10 mg.

Pyridoxine Hydrochloride, U.S.P., is a constituent of an enzyme which plays a role in amino-acid metabolism in contrast to most of the other parts of the 'B complex' which are essential parts of various factors concerned with carbohydrate metabolism. It may be given in the treatment of morning sickness during pregnancy and irradiation sickness after X-ray and similar therapies of cancer. Dosage is not critically established, usually 25–100 mg. per day, which may well be more than is necessary.

ANTI-ANAEMIA FACTORS

It was discovered by Minot and Murphy in 1926 that a rapid and striking improvement can be effected in the condition of patients suffering from pernicious anaemia if liver be added to their diet in sufficient amounts. This disease (in contradistinction to simple anaemias, p. 66) is characterized by a great reduction in the number of the red cells, but each red cell has usually its full complement of haemoglobin. The disease is not due to lack of iron, and the administration of iron is of no remedial value in it. When a sufficient amount of liver is taken in the diet, the number of red blood corpuscles rapidly increases, and the symptoms resulting from this poverty disappear. Usually within a week of commencement of treatment, there occurs a characteristic increase in the number of reticulocytes in the blood which reaches a maximum about the tenth day, after which their number falls again about equally rapidly. Following this, at the end of about a fortnight, the significant rise in the number of red cells begins. If degenerative changes have already occurred in the central nervous system in pernicious anaemia they can only be checked by treatment with liver.

The amount of liver necessary to maintain health is so great ($\frac{1}{4}$–$\frac{1}{2}$ lb. per day) as to be intolerable and relapse of the disease occurs if liver is discontinued. For a long time the active principle defied extraction and purification and use had to be made of injections of liver extract. The picture became clearer when it was realized, largely as a result of the work of Castle, that two factors were needed in association—an extrinsic factor in foods and stored in the liver, the anti-anaemia factor, and an intrinsic factor evolved by the pyloric mucosa and necessary for absorption of the former. Pernicious anaemia is a deficiency disease of this area of mucosa, one of its characteristic signs being absence of gastric acid (histamine fast). The logical treatment is to replace this deficiency by administering the intrinsic factor and a full diet, as is done when **Powdered Stomach**, U.S.P., is used. Unfortunately this is an impure and nauseating preparation.

Cyanocobalamin, B.P., U.S.P., (Vitamin B_{12}). In 1948 a red crystalline substance was isolated from liver and provisionally called Vitamin B_{12}. It is now more conveniently obtained commercially from the fermentation liquors of *Streptomyces* *griseus.* Its exact composition is known. It contains cobalt and has the official name of cyanocobalamin.

Cyanocobalamin appears to be the main anti-anaemic principle of liver and is as effective in the treatment of pernicious anaemia and subacute combined degeneration of the spinal cord as liver extract. Cyanocobalamin is cheaper than the liver extract, more constant in activity, and does not give rise to allergic complications as liver extract sometimes does. It has no effect orally (unless exceptionally and in very large doses) as it does not contain the intrinsic factor which is necessary for its absorption from the alimentary canal. Doses, by intramuscular injection: initial dose, 50–100 micrograms; maintenance dose, 50–100 micrograms every two or three weeks. The U.S.P. contains *Vitamin B₁₂ with Intrinsic Factor Concentrate,* a yellowish powdered extract of hog stomach reinforced with cyanocobalamin, which, being taken by mouth, provides both elements of the anti-anaemia complex.

Folic Acid, B.P., U.S.P., another member of the Vitamin B complex which has been isolated and synthesized, was originally obtained from spinach and other green leaves, whence its name. Folic acid has been used in the treatment of pernicious anaemia and other macrocytic anaemias, in which it stimulates erythropoiesis. It has the advantages over liver extracts (p. 233) that it is effective when given by mouth and in small doses, and it materially reduces the cost and inconvenience of treatment. It does not prevent the degenerative changes in the nervous system that often occur in pernicious anaemia. Indeed in some cases it appears to induce them and they may disappear again when pteroylglutamic (folic) acid is replaced by cyanocobalamin. It is now considered to have no place in the therapy of true pernicious anaemia but is of value in the megalocytic anaemias of pregnancy and sprue. It is given by mouth, dose 5–20 mg. daily.

VITAMIN C

That the disease called scurvy (which was especially liable to occur in sailors when, on long voyages, they had to live on salted meat without fresh fruit or vegetables) could be cured by administration of orange or lemon juice has been known for two centuries. So far as organic factors are concerned, this was the first indication of the necessity of certain accessory food factors in the diet and of the possibility of curing the ailments due to their deficiency. In 1933 it was shown that the substance responsible for this curative effect in scurvy was ascorbic acid, a compound related to glucose and which had provisionally been called Vitamin C.

Serious lack of ascorbic acid in the diet leads to increased fragility of the capillaries, due to deficiency of the intercellular material, with consequent liability to haemorrhages in various tissues, especially in the gums, periosteum, and joints. There occur also defective development of the bones and teeth and probably a diminished resistance to certain infections.

Ascorbic Acid, B.P., U.S.P., is a colourless, crystalline solid, soluble in water. Rich natural sources are oranges, lemons, blackcurrants, and tomatoes. Green vegetables, e.g. cabbage, contain it, but it is easily destroyed by cooking, and it cannot be stored in the body, being rapidly excreted in the urine. An optimum daily requirement is about 50 mg., and many diets furnish much less than this. In infancy and old age, during pregnancy and lactation, it is important that the supply of Vitamin C should be adequate.

An average dose is 50 mg., but 250 mg. may be given in scurvy. There seems to be no danger from overdosage.

VITAMIN D

Clinical observation had led to the opinion that the disease rickets, which was common in ill-nourished children, was improved both by administration of cod-liver oil and by exposure to sunlight before any relation was known to exist between these two, apparently disconnected, remedial influences. Rickets is now known to be due to lack of Vitamin D in the diet. Several different but related substances, all derived from sterols, can cure rickets and may be included under the term Vitamin D. For therapeutic purposes the most important are

Calciferol, B.P., U.S.P., (Vitamin D_2 or viosterol) and *Activated 7-Dehydrocholesterol*, U.S.P., (Vitamin D_3), both of which are formed from inactive provitamins by the action of ultra-violet light. Calciferol is obtained from ergosterol, a sterol found in yeast, and is made artificially by exposure of this to light. It does not occur in fish oils.

Vitamin D_3 can be obtained from irradiated 7-dihydro-cholesterol and occurs naturally in fish oils, milk, &c. The con-version of an inactive, into an active, sterol occurs in the skin under the influence of sunlight. The value of cod-liver oil and sunlight in the treatment of rickets has now received a rational explanation; the former cures because it contains an active vitamin, the latter because it effects a stage in the conversion of inactive provitamin into an active vitamin.

Rickets is a disease characterized especially by deformities of the bones and teeth, due to defective calcification. Vitamin D increases the absorption of calcium from the gut and diminishes its excretion through the mucous membrane into the lumen of the large intestine. The calcium in the blood is increased and the bones and teeth receive their normal requirements. Infants are most susceptible to rickets, and the amount of Vitamin D in milk depends upon the amount of exposure to sunlight of the animal supplying the milk. A disease, osteomalacia, which occurs in adults, especially pregnant women, is also due to calcium deficiency and may be cured by Vitamin D. Overdosage with Vitamin D may cause an excessive absorption of calcium phosphate with calcification in the aorta, kidneys, &c.

The official preparations of Vitamins A and D may be con-sidered together, as both are soluble in fats and occur in the most readily available natural sources of them, viz. fish oils.

Cod-liver oil is a fixed oil extracted from the fresh liver of the cod (*Gadus morrhua*). It has a pale yellow colour and a slight but rather disagreeable odour. It is an easily absorbable fat and is therefore a valuable food apart from its vitamin content, and has long been used, mainly from this point of view, in malnu-trition and wasting diseases, such as tuberculosis. It has now acquired a new importance from the recognition of its high vitamin content, especially of Vitamins A and D. Each gramme of *Cod-liver Oil*, B.P., U.S.P. should contain at least 600 International Units of Vitamin A and 85 I.U. of Vitamin D. The U.S.P. contains also *Oleovitamins A*, and *D*, separately, which may consist of a suitable fish-liver oil or suitable sources of Vitamins A and D dissolved in a vegetable oil. They can be used as a substitute for cod-liver oil. *Halibut-Liver Oil* contains in 1 G. 30,000 I.U. of Vitamin A (and usually, though in the B.P. not compulsorily, about 3,000 Units of Vitamin D). It is an especially rich source of Vitamin A. *Calciferol*, B.P., U.S.P., (Vitamin D_2), contains 40,000 Units of antirachitic activity in 1 milligram, and can more conveniently be given as the *Solution of Calciferol*, which contains 3,000 Units of Vitamin D in 1 gramme.

The optimum dosage of vitamins depends upon the degree and duration of the deficiency. For full health and development the animal requires a regular and definite amount of certain vitamins, and this amount, if not forthcoming in the diet, should be made up by supplementary administration. From the point of view of preventing the ill effects of deficiency, the dose required is called the prophylactic dose. Larger doses, so-called therapeutic doses, are required to cure established effects due to serious deficiency. It may be taken as a rough guide that the daily requirements for an adult are about 5,000 International Units of Vitamin A and 500 I.U. of Vitamin D. Growing children and pregnant women require rather more, and much larger doses may be given therapeutically for a limited time.

Two other vitamins, additional to those mentioned above, are believed, so far as present knowledge goes, to be of therapeutic importance in man.

VITAMIN E

This occurs especially in vegetable oils like wheat-germ oil and is a compound, α-tocopherol, which has been isolated and synthesized. Female animals deprived of Vitamin E may conceive, but the embryos are resorbed or aborted. Young rats deficient in this vitamin develop paralysis of the hind limbs. These findings have suggested its use in habitual or threatened abortion and in certain nervous diseases, but the therapeutic value, if any, of Vitamin E in human disease is still in the experimental stage.

VITAMIN K

Chickens fed on a diet deficient in fat may develop a fatal haemorrhagic tendency, due to a decrease in plasma prothrombin. This is due to lack of Vitamin K, which is soluble in fats and for the absorption of which bile is necessary. In obstructive jaundice, the clotting of blood may be delayed owing to lack of bile in the gut with the consequent diminished absorption of Vitamin K, and there is a tendency to haemorrhages. This can be checked by administration of Vitamin K, which is also of value in haemorrhagic disease of the new-born. This vitamin is a derivative of naphthoquinone, and synthetic derivatives having similar activities are available.

Menaphthone, B.P., 1–5 mg., *Menadione,* U.S.P., 1 mg., is the most important of these. Being more active than Vitamin K and easily made synthetically it is usually employed in Vitamin K deficiency. Menaphthone is almost insoluble in water and the B.P. has an oily *Injection* for intramuscular use. In combination with sodium bisulphite it is freely soluble and the U.S.P. has *Menadione Sodium Bisulfite*, which may be given intramuscularly or intravenously.

The development and widespread use of coumarin anticoagulants which act by antagonizing Vitamin K has brought about a greatly increased need for suitable Vitamin K preparations to deal with cases of overdosage by these substances. A dose of 50–100 mg. of the soluble salt of Menadione may be needed to restore prothrombin levels (p. 209).

Menadiol Sodium Diphosphate, U.S.P., is a water soluble dihydro derivative of menadione. It may be given by all usual routes of administration in doses of 3–6 mg. daily and is valuable in a dose of 75 mg. given intramuscularly as an antidote to dicoumeral poisoning.

The natural vitamin is a naphthoquinone and is available

as **Phytonadione**, U.S.P. It is a liquid, insoluble in water and is quicker, more potent, and more prolonged in its activity than the synthetic analogues mentioned. Some 250–500 mg. may be given orally, or in emergency by slow intravenous injection at the rate of 10 mg. per minute of an emulsion, as a counter to over-zealous anticoagulant therapy.

XX

PHENOL AND ALLIED AROMATIC COMPOUNDS

NUMEROUS derivatives of benzene are used in medicine either for their local actions as antiseptics or for their actions as analgesics or antipyretics. Benzene itself, C_6H_6, is not so active as many of its derivatives, partly because of its insolubility, but chiefly from the difficulty with which it combines with protoplasm; but relatively slight changes in its composition may produce a great increase in its physiological activity, such as the substitution of —OH for —H, forming phenol. The benzene ring itself is not easily decomposed in the body, and for the most part passes through it unchanged, though the organism does possess the power of destroying the benzene ring of those aromatic amino-acids which enter into the composition of proteins. Foreign aromatic compounds require to be rendered innocuous by being combined with sulphuric acid to form aromatic sulphates, or with glycocoll to form acids of the type of hippuric acid. The few exceptions are compounds which so closely resemble the protein fractions in their structure that they fall victims with these to the normal destructive processes.

PHENOL

Phenol (Carbolic Acid) C_6H_5OH, was the first substance intentionally used as an antiseptic, its earliest use by Lister dating back to 1867. It forms colourless crystals, which may become pinkish on keeping, with a characteristic smell and pungent sweetish taste, soluble 1 in 13 in water. The presence of the hydroxyl group renders phenol more soluble than benzol and more reactive with protoplasm. Phenol forms a loose combination with proteins and is also more soluble in lipoids than in water, so that it readily penetrates cells. It is a general protoplasmic poison, killing all living cells if in sufficient concentration.

EXTERNAL ACTIONS. When concentrated, phenol is a powerful caustic. Solutions even so dilute as 2 per cent., if applied to the skin and prevented from evaporating, may cause local gangrene. This occurs most readily in the case of the fingers. The epidermis becomes at first white, wrinkled, and opaque, and at least partly anaesthetic, and later necrotic. It is therefore dangerous to keep a wet phenol dressing on the fingers, as local gangrene may occur even within 24 hours. As an antiseptic phenol has now been superseded. It is irritant to wounds or mucous membranes in the concentrations needed to inhibit bacterial growth, and it is fairly easily absorbed from any absorbing surface, and thus may produce general poisoning. Its ready absorbability renders it useless as an intestinal antiseptic. Its most common use now is to keep instruments sterile.

ACTIONS AFTER ABSORPTION. Phenol is readily absorbed. It is not now used therapeutically for any action that it can exert after absorption, and poisoning with it is now uncommon, so that only a brief reference to the effects of large doses is needed. It has no high degree of selective action, so that most tissues are more or less injured by it. The central nervous system is markedly affected, being depressed, with or without a previous stage of excitation. Especially with large poisonous doses in man, coma and death may occur in less than an hour, with no preceding convulsive stage. There is usually a rapid fall of temperature. Respiratory failure is the main cause of death, but the heart and vasomotor centre are also depressed.

Phenol is excreted in the urine partly as such and partly oxidized to dioxy- compounds. All these compounds are excreted in combination with either sulphuric or glycuronic acid. The presence of these compounds may give to the urine a smoky colour, which darkens further on standing, owing to further oxidation.

The entrance of alkyl groups into the nucleus diminishes the general toxicity without proportionately diminishing the antiseptic power, e.g. in cresol, $C_6H_4 \cdot OH \cdot CH_3$. Owing to this, substances of the cresol type have largely replaced phenol itself as antiseptics, because an equal antiseptic action can be obtained by them with greater safety. But this introduction of an alkyl group, while diminishing the toxicity, has the disadvantage that it diminishes also the solubility. They are in fact not sufficiently soluble to be used as surgical antiseptics in simple solution, but have to be emulsified in some way. A preparation like *Solution of Cresol with Soap*, B.P., which is used as a surgical antiseptic, contains cresols emulsified by means of soft soap.

In compounds of this type the substitution of Cl to replace H in the benzene ring may still further increase antiseptic activity. *Chlorocresol*, B.P., (*parachlorometacresol*), is used especially for preserving fluids for parenteral injection. The corresponding xylenol compound, *Chloroxylenol*, B.P., is even more actively antiseptic. Preparations containing it, dissolved with the aid of soap, are claimed to be less irritant and less toxic, for an equal degree of antiseptic action, than other phenolic antiseptics. The *Solution of Chloroxylenol*, B.P., is such a preparation.

Hexachlorophene, U.S.P., is a more elaborate chlorinated hydroxyphenol compound which is insoluble in water. It is incorporated in soaps, creams, &c., for topical application from which it is adsorbed into the skin. There it continues for some time to inhibit the growth of micro-organisms.

The substances of the foregoing group, including phenol itself, can be obtained by fractional distillation of tars or can be made synthetically. *Tar*, B.P., (Wood Tar), and *Prepared Coal Tar*, B.P., *Coal Tar*, U.S.P., contain a variety of phenol derivatives and are used as antiseptics, especially for the skin.

In the foregoing paragraphs the modifications in the action of phenol brought about by the introduction of alkyl groups have been considered. Brief reference must now be made to the introduction of hydroxyl groups. As already pointed out, the entrance of a hydroxyl group into the benzene nucleus makes it more soluble and physiologically more active than benzene itself. The addition of further hydroxyl groups usually makes the resulting substance still more toxic. Dihydroxybenzenes generally resemble phenol in action but are more poisonous. One of them, *Resorcinol*, B.P., U.S.P., is sometimes used in ointments for skin diseases. *Hexylresorcinol*, U.S.P., is a more powerful antiseptic and has been used as such, externally for the skin and mucous membranes and internally especially in infections of the urinary tract (p. 290). It is also used as an anthelmintic (p. 307).

VOLATILE OILS

Many other aromatic compounds, more or less closely resembling phenol in constitution and action, have been used medicinally. One group of these, which resembles phenol fairly closely, is that of the volatile or essential oils. They are aromatic compounds and have no chemical relation to the fixed oils, which they resemble only in their solubilities. They can be distilled unchanged, and are usually obtained from plants by distillation, whereas a fixed oil so treated splits into its two components, glycerin and a fatty acid.

The characteristic odour of plants is generally due to the presence, in the flower or elsewhere, of a volatile oil. Volatile oils are, therefore, very widely distributed in the vegetable kingdom, and, as plants containing them would often attract attention from their pleasant smell, a very large number of such plants have come into culinary and medicinal use, owing such action as they have almost entirely to the volatile oil in them.

While the volatile oils differ from one another in composition, as a result of which they differ in smell and, to some extent, in pharmacological action, they nevertheless have a generic resemblance in chemical structure and in action.

Most of them are of the nature of terpenes, having the formula $C_{10}H_{16}$. They are usually just sufficiently soluble (of the order 1 in 5,000) in water to impart their odour to it. They are antiseptics, but too insoluble and too expensive for general use. They usually irritate the skin in concentration, especially if evaporation be prevented, but after the preliminary irritation some of them produce partial local anaesthesia like phenol.

Taken internally, they stimulate appetite, especially if the odour is agreeable. They aid in the expulsion of gas from the stomach and tend to prevent colic, apparently by suppressing excessive contractions of the gut. In medicinal doses they have little action while circulating in the blood. They are excreted in the urine, usually combined with glycuronic acid, or in the lungs unchanged, and especially in the former exert a mild antiseptic action. Like a great many mild irritants they increase the secretion of urine while passing through the kidney.

Larger doses affect chiefly the central nervous system, and here the actions of individual oils vary. Usually they depress the central nervous system eventually, but some of them, e.g. absinthe, first stimulate the cerebral centres and may even produce convulsions. Their action on the central nervous system is therefore not unlike that of phenol.

It remains here only to mention which particular oils have come to be used for the various actions that they all exert more or less.

1. Flavouring agents. Of these, oils of anise, caraway, cinnamon, clove, coriander, lemon, and peppermint may be mentioned. The usual dose of the pure oils is 0·06–0·2 ml. (1–3 min.). Some of them have, as an official preparation, a *Concentrated Water*, e.g. **Concentrated Peppermint Water**, B.P., which is a solution of the oil in alcohol and water, and is used mainly for flavouring mixtures in doses of 0·3–1 ml. (5–15 min.).

2. Some are used as counter-irritants, e.g. **Turpentine Oil** in the form of **Liniment of Turpentine**, B.P. (p. 132).

3. Many of them can be used as carminatives (p. 43), that is, to aid in the expulsion of gases from the stomach. This they do apparently by relaxing the cardiac orifice of the stomach. They are very commonly used to prevent griping by relaxing spasmodic contractions of the gut. Many purgative and astringent pills and powders contain a volatile oil to prevent colic. In the purgative preparations the volatile oil prevents the colic which might be set up by the purgative which is being prescribed; in the astringent preparations it prevents the colic which is an accompaniment of the diarrhoea that is being treated. The

household use of Dill Water, for the relief of griping in infants, may be mentioned.

4. Of the oils especially useful for imparting a pleasant odour to preparations may be mentioned oils of lavender, rose, and rosemary.

5. Probably all of the volatile oils exert some diuretic action. Oil of juniper was formerly used specifically for this purpose. The superiority of gin, which is flavoured with oil of juniper, as a diuretic over other alcoholic beverages has been long recognized.

STEAROPTENES

Under certain circumstances crystalline substances separate out from the volatile oils. Three of these, thymol, camphor, and menthol, called stearoptenes and containing oxygen in their molecule, are of considerable medicinal importance. Chemically and pharmacologically they very closely resemble the volatile oils proper.

Thymol, B.P., U.S.P., is a powerful antiseptic used chiefly for the nose and mouth. It is sparingly soluble in water, freely soluble in alcohol.

Camphor, B.P., U.S.P., is a less efficient antiseptic. Locally it is used chiefly as a counter-irritant (p. 132) in the form of *Liniment of Camphor*, B.P., (Camphorated Oil), a solution of 1 part in 4 of a fixed oil. Camphor has long been used in the East as a 'stimulant'. Taken internally it produces a sensation of warmth in the stomach, such as is produced by other gastric irritants like alcohol or mustard. Larger doses stimulate the central nervous system, and may produce restlessness, excitement, delirium, and even epileptiform convulsions. Those effects are not of course produced by medicinal doses, but they may afford some explanation for the use of camphor, especially in the East, as a stimulant and aphrodisiac.

Camphor has been widely used as a stimulant to the circulation. Pharmacological evidence has failed to disclose any direct stimulant action on a normal heart, but it is claimed that camphor may have such an action when the heart muscle is depressed. There are more certain grounds for believing that it may stimulate the vasomotor centre. This is part of its general stimulative action on the central nervous system. This uncertainty of action of camphor has prompted the search for more reliable synthetic stimulants, e.g. leptazol (p. 81).

Menthol, B.P., U.S.P., generally resembles thymol and camphor in action. If rubbed into the skin, it produces a local sensation of cold followed by partial local anaesthesia. The sensation of cold is supposed to be due to stimulation of the terminations of the nerves that convey the sensation of cold, and the anaesthesia to paralysis of the touch and pain nerves. Almost the only medicinal use of menthol is for this local effect. It is rubbed on the skin for headache and neuralgia, which it sometimes relieves. Inhalations of menthol have a local anaesthetic action on the mucous membranes of the upper air passages and may relieve pain and cough in laryngitis.

XXI

DRUGS USED IN BACTERIAL INFECTIONS

LOCAL ANTISEPTICS

IN previous chapters drugs have been considered primarily from the standpoint of their actions on various organs in man, and with a view to explaining the remedial effects that they can produce in disease. A great many diseases are due to parasitic organisms, and many examples have already been incidentally given of drugs which exert, among other actions, a destructive effect on pathogenic organisms. For example, phenol, mercury, and arsenic all have important therapeutic uses dependent upon some parasiticidal action, but, for reasons of convenience, their general actions have been discussed elsewhere. We may now consider drugs rather from the point of view of their actions upon parasites themselves, classifying them according to the type of infection for which they are chiefly used.

It will be readily intelligible that the problem of treating infective diseases will depend not only on the type of micro-organism but on the site of the infection. A particular bacterium may infect the skin, the larynx, the lungs, or the peritoneum, and the same chemical agent may not be equally applicable to each of these situations. It will be possible here only to give a brief résumé of the more important drugs which are used in the treatment of infections, and to give some indication of the type of infections for which they are chiefly used.

The deliberate use of chemical agents for destroying pathogenic micro-organisms began with Lister, who first recorded his observations in 1867. He was primarily concerned with the prevention of suppuration, putrefaction, or 'sepsis' in wounds, and chemical agents such as phenol, which were employed to prevent such suppuration, were called antiseptics. When the work of Pasteur, Koch, and their successors showed that a very large number of diseases are due to infection by different micro-organisms, the use of chemical agents to control such infections was extended far beyond their first use to control suppuration in wounds. Though the word 'antiseptic' is still used in its original sense of a substance which will diminish sepsis, it may now be more generally defined as a drug which inhibits the growth of micro-organisms. If the latter are actually killed, the drug is called a disinfectant.

Pathogenic organisms can be divided into a few broad classes. To a certain extent treatment of infections of each of these groups involves different problems and is often subserved by different groups of remedies.

Bacteria, which include bacilli and cocci, are minute uni-cellular organisms which are generally regarded as belonging to the vegetable kingdom. They give rise not only to superficial and localized infections of the skin, wounds, and mucous membranes, &c., but also to deep infections, e.g. of the lungs, peritoneum, or even of the blood itself. In some of these cases it is comparatively easy to control infection by the aid of antiseptics; in other cases it may be difficult or impossible. Some bacteria are much more easily killed than others, and spore forms are as a rule unusually resistant.

The antiseptic action of a drug can be tested by determining what concentration of it is necessary to arrest the growth of bacteria in a culture medium. So tested, a very large number of substances could be labelled as antiseptics, but only a very few of these are of any practical value in the treatment of infections. A micro-organism is killed by some chemical interaction between it and the antiseptic, but the same interaction will be liable to take place between the antiseptic and other cells which more or less resemble the micro-organism in composition. The practical problem is, therefore, to find an antiseptic which will check the growth of bacteria without seriously damaging the cells of the tissues. This problem would probably be in most cases insoluble were it not for the natural defensive mechanisms of the body against bacterial invasion. These are in continual operation, and are, in the aggregate, of far greater value than any antiseptic. In spite of the omnipresence of pathogenic bacteria, many wounds healed spontaneously before antiseptics were introduced, and they do so now. Clearly, therefore, it is of the utmost importance not to interfere with the local or general defensive mechanisms of the body. The broad principle underlying the employment of antiseptics is to assist these mechanisms in the battle against bacterial invasion. It follows that it is not necessary that the antiseptic should kill the bacteria. If the vitality of bacteria is diminished below a certain point, the natural defensive reactions of the body, e.g. phagocytosis or antitoxin formation, are fortunately as a rule adequate to repel the bacterial invasion. It is chiefly owing to this co-operation that, especially in superficial infections of wounds or mucous membranes, a concentration of an antiseptic which will not seriously injure the tissues themselves may be effective in inhibiting the multiplication of bacteria. On the other hand, when the bacteria are of high virulence or difficult to kill, or when they invade inaccessible regions or vital organs, all the means at present at our disposal may be inadequate to protect life.

An important distinction must be drawn between local (superficial) and systemic (general) antiseptics. If an antiseptic can reach an organ, e.g. the lungs or kidney, only by being carried to it by the blood stream, or if the infection involve the blood itself, then all the organs of the body will be subjected to the action of the antiseptic. This will not happen to the same extent if the antiseptic be applied to a surface such as the skin or conjunctiva, or at all if the antiseptic be not absorbed from that surface. It is often true, therefore, that an antiseptic can be used for direct or local application to a surface which will be inadmissible as a remote antiseptic. Yet other disinfectants may be used for disinfecting rooms, clothing, or surgical instruments, for here no question of general or local toxic action of the antiseptic on the tissues need arise. In this chapter some of the more important local antiseptics will be mentioned. The problems of systemic antiseptics (Chap. XXIV) can be best understood after a more general consideration of Chemotherapy (Chap. XXIII).

So far as superficial infections are concerned, the same type of antiseptic may be applicable, for example, to a wound, a mucous membrane, or the skin, though even here certain antiseptics are more suitable for one region than for another.

Of antiseptics generally used for surface application which have previously been considered may be mentioned ethyl alcohol, the phenol group, and the heavy metals. Some other antiseptics can conveniently be dealt with here.

Boric Acid, B.P., U.S.P., has a feeble disinfectant action, and is generally capable merely of restraining bacterial growth. It is widely used as a dusting powder, alone or diluted. It is also used in solution as a wash for catarrh of mucous membranes, e.g. in conjunctivitis (2–4 per cent.). *Ointment of Boric Acid*, B.P. (1·0 per cent.), is used as a mild skin antiseptic.

Chlorine is the active antiseptic in a variety of preparations. It acts as an antiseptic by uniting with the proteins of bacteria; but as it combines also with proteins of the tissues, it tends to be rapidly used up, so that the antiseptic action is transient. Chlorine is commonly employed in the form of hypochlorous acid or a hypochlorite which readily gives off chlorine. *Surgical Solution of Chlorinated Soda*, B.P., is one such solution.

Chloramine, B.P., is a compound which contains about 12 per cent. of active chlorine. It forms white, almost odourless crystals, soluble 1 in 7 in water. It is less irritating than hypochlorous acid and does not give off its chlorine so rapidly. It is used in 0·1 to 2 per cent. aqueous solution for wounds or mucous membranes.

Iodine, B.P., acts as an antiseptic in much the same way as chlorine. Iodine forms dark crystals with a metallic lustre, a distinctive odour, and an acrid taste. It is feebly soluble in water, soluble in solutions of iodides or in alcohol. It is an irritant, and *Strong Solution of Iodine*, B.P., may be used for counter-irritation (p. 130). *Weak Solution of Iodine*, B.P. (2·5 per cent.), or *Iodine Tincture*, U.S.P. (2 per cent.), are used for their antiseptic action, for example, for the skin, tonsils, or abrasions.

Alcoholic solutions of iodine (2–5 per cent.) are frequently used to sterilize the skin before operations, both iodine and alcohol acting as antiseptics. The iodine stains the skin light brown, but this is in some ways an advantage as it shows up the area to which the solution has been applied.

Many dyes are powerful antiseptics and several have been used as such. Some of these are derivatives of triphenylmethane, of which one of the best-known is *Crystal Violet* (Gentian Violet), B.P., U.S.P. This dye stains Gram-positive bacteria and has a selective antiseptic action on them. *Brilliant Green*, B.P., is related chemically to crystal violet and has similar actions. These dyes have been used in solutions for the treatment of wounds, ulcers, burns, &c.

Proflavine Hemisulphate, B.P., an acridine derivative, has been widely used as an antiseptic for wounds. It develops its antiseptic action slowly, but that action is not so much impeded by the presence of serum as is the case with many antiseptics. Proflavine is less toxic and less irritant to the tissues than acriflavine.

Aminacrine Hydrochloride, B.P., a colourless acridine derivative is much used in an antiseptic cream for obstetrical work.

Certain dyes, used for medicinal purposes other than as antiseptics, may be briefly mentioned here. *Methylene Blue*, B.P., has been used as a local antiseptic and also has some remedial effect in malaria. It is excreted in the urine and can be used as a test for renal efficiency; *Indigo Carmine*, B.P., can also be used for this purpose (p. 313). Scarlet Red is used to stimulate the growth of epithelium.

OXIDIZING AGENTS

Certain oxidizing agents are used as antiseptics, the most important being peroxide of hydrogen and potassium permanganate. They act by liberating oxygen which unites with proteins of bacteria and also with tissue proteins. All the available oxygen is soon given up and the antiseptic action exhausted.

Hydrogen Peroxide, (H_2O_2), is used in the form of a 6 per cent. *Solution of Hydrogen Peroxide*, B.P. Each volume of this solution contains twenty volumes of available oxygen. The *Hydrogen Peroxide Solution*, U.S.P., contains 3 per cent. of H_2O_2. It gives off this oxygen very rapidly in contact with living tissues and especially with pus or blood. In addition to its bactericidal action, hydrogen peroxide has a singular value in loosening and disintegrating and bringing to the surface pus or infective material in wound or cavities. This it does mechanically by the effervescence of oxygen.

Potassium Permanganate, B.P., U.S.P., ($KMnO_4$), forms dark purple prismatic crystals, odourless, soluble 1 in 16 in water. It liberates oxygen too slowly to produce the mechanical effect of peroxide of hydrogen. It is used chiefly as an antiseptic for mucous membranes, especially of the urethra, mouth, or throat. It is occasionally used for the skin, which it colours brown. It has been tried as a chemical antidote to many poisons, e.g. by stomach in morphine poisoning or locally in snakebite, but is not very effective.

Formaldehyde ($H \cdot CHO$) is an irritant gas which is used as *Solution of Formaldehyde*, B.P., U.S.P., or as a vapour for disinfecting rooms, clothing, instruments, &c.

DETERGENTS

The word 'detergent' means primarily a 'cleansing agent'. Many chemical substances are used for this purpose which they achieve mainly by lowering surface tension, whereby they may produce a variety of effects, e.g. wetting, foaming, deflocculation, emulsification. They now have important and varied uses in many industries in addition to their medical uses.

ANIONIC DETERGENTS. The oldest and best-known detergents are soaps, potassium or sodium salts of one or more fatty acids. The surface activity of a detergent depends upon certain properties residing in its molecular structure, which can be illustrated by a simple soap like sodium stearate, $C_{17}H_{35}COO^-Na^+$. The anion contains a long hydrocarbon chain $C_{17}H_{35}$, which is water-repellent and oil-soluble, and COO^-, a water-attracting and water-soluble polar group which confers water-solubility on the whole compound. At an oil–water interface molecules of this type orientate themselves so that the water-soluble group stays in the water surface while the hydrocarbon chain moves into the oil. This leads to a reduction in surface tension. When, as in a soap, the long chain is part of the anion, the substance is called an anion-active or anionic detergent. One such is *Sodium Lauryl Sulphate*, B.P., U.S.P.

CATIONIC DETERGENTS. The most important of these are quaternary ammonium compounds with a type structure $R—N(CH_3)_3^+ Cl^-$, one valency of ammonium being occupied by a long-chain fatty acid R, the other three by methyl or similar groups, the anion being either chlorine or bromine. They act in a similar way to a soap, the hydrocarbon chain being oil-soluble, the nitrogen portion of the molecule water-soluble. In this case, however, the long chain is contained in the cation, and the substance called a cation-active or cationic detergent. Cationic detergents are incompatible with anionic detergents such as soap. They are absorbed on to the surface of bacteria and are bacteriostatic in weak, and bactericidal in stronger solutions. They are extensively used in domestic and hospital hygiene to remove grease, dirt, and microbes from utensils and clothing. They are particularly effective against Gram-positive organisms, but ineffective against spores, fungi, and viruses, and are not injurious to delicate surfaces. One such is *Cetrimide*, B.P., others are *Benzalkonium Chloride*, U.S.P., and *Benzethonium Chloride*, U.S.P. They are used in solution to disinfect skin, to treat superficial injuries, and to irrigate mucous surfaces.

FUNGISTATIC AGENTS

The antifungal activity of salicylic acid has already been mentioned. Probably this is largely due to its keratolytic property which removes the dead skin in which the superficial infection flourishes. Various dyes, benzoic acid, iodine, phenyl-mercuric nitrate and thiomersal (an organic mercurial antiseptic) have powers of controlling fungal infections of the skin. It must be remembered that there are many species of pathogenic fungi and it is not to be expected that any one antifungal agent will be effective against them all. One member of the series of unsaturated fatty acids, *Undecylenic Acid*, U.S.P., (Undecenoic Acid), is widely used for these infections, e.g. athlete's foot. It is a yellow liquid with a characteristic unpleasant odour, insoluble in water, applied as a cream, ointment, or emulsion.

LOCAL USE OF ANTISEPTICS

Of those mentioned, the following must be regarded merely as a few examples of antiseptics which have been found suitable for certain localities. For sterilizing the skin prior to operations, ethyl alcohol, detergents, or solutions of iodine or of proflavine are frequently employed. A great variety of antiseptics are used in skin diseases and generally applied in the form of ointments, e.g. boric acid, salicylic acid, zinc oxide, mercury compounds. For mucous membranes, which are usually sensitive, irritating antiseptics must be avoided. For the conjunctiva solutions of boric acid, zinc sulphate, or protein compounds of silver are largely used, and for the urethra solutions of potassium permanganate, silver protein, or zinc sulphate. Peroxide of hydrogen and chlorine compounds are favourite antiseptics for wounds. In recent years, however, penicillin and other antibiotics, though their chief use is as systemic antiseptics, have been widely used also as local antiseptics.

XXII

ANTITOXINS, VACCINES, AND TOXINS

A. PASSIVE IMMUNIZATION

ANTITOXINS

THE great importance of the natural defensive reactions of the body against bacterial invasion must briefly be mentioned. One of these reactions consists in the formation by the tissues of 'antibodies' which are shed into the blood and body fluids and which tend to inactivate bacteria or their toxins. When a foreign protein ('antigen') is injected into an animal it provokes the formation of an 'antibody', which is specific for that particular protein. This reaction occurs to all injected proteins and to proteins mainly. It does not occur when they are given by mouth, because the proteins are broken down in the alimentary canal and absorbed chiefly as amino-acids, which do not provoke this reaction. The amino-acids absorbed from the food can be re-synthesized into proteins natural to the animal, and antibody-formation would appear to be designed to prevent the entrance and continued existence of foreign proteins in the blood or tissues. Ordinary digestion prevents this occurring with the proteins of the food.

In ordinary life there is little opportunity of foreign proteins entering the blood or tissues in an unaltered state unless conveyed by bacteria or protozoa, so that, for our limited purpose here, antibody-formation can be regarded as of importance chiefly as being one of the most important natural mechanisms for resisting invasion of bacteria, or for neutralizing the protein-like poisons or toxins which they produce. It is perhaps the most general method by which a bacterial disease is overcome and 'immunity' to it acquired.

In a disease like diphtheria, for example, the injury to the patient occurs chiefly in two ways: in the first place from the mechanical and other effects of the bacterial growth on the upper air passages or elsewhere, and secondly as the result of the toxins formed by the bacteria which are absorbed and are powerful poisons for the heart and nervous system. Natural cure of the disease results largely from the formation of antibodies which inhibit bacterial multiplication or neutralize their toxins. If the bacterial infection be severe or if the patient have a low resistance to it, this antibody-formation will not take place to a sufficient degree or sufficiently rapidly to save the patient from the effects of the toxin. Once the toxin has combined with the heart or nervous system, antitoxin is then incapable of dislodging or neutralizing it. It would clearly be of advantage, therefore, if the patient could be supplied with the necessary antitoxin, especially before the toxin has had time to exert its injurious effects. This can be done by injecting antitoxin obtained from a horse which has been immunized to diphtheria toxin.

The procedure adopted is briefly as follows. Diphtheria toxin is first obtained from the filtrate of a broth culture of diphtheria bacillus. A horse is immunized by repeated injections (at four-day intervals) of the toxin, the dose being gradually increased according to the amount of reaction. Injections are given from four to six months until the blood acquires a sufficiently high antitoxic power. The horse is then bled to the amount of perhaps 10 litres, and the separated serum collected. The serum may be used as such, or the globulins, which contain practically all the antitoxin, can be separated by fractional precipitation from the other serum proteins and used in saline solution. This antitoxic serum must be standardized according to its power of neutralizing diphtheria toxin, and this power is expressed in terms of 'Units' compared with a standard antitoxin.

Diphtheria Antitoxin, B.P., should possess in its liquid forms a potency of not less than 500 Units per millilitre. It is of great value both as a prophylactic and as a curative agent against diphtheria. Its value depends upon its being given early and in adequate doses. The protective dose may be 500–2,000 Units, the curative dose not less than 10,000 Units, by injection, B.P., 20,000 Units, U.S.P.

Tetanus Antitoxin is prepared in a similar way from the serum of a horse immunized to tetanus toxin. It is of great value as a protective against tetanus, dose B.P. not less than 1,500 Units; and of some, though much less, value when tetanus has developed, in which case the dose has to be much larger, not less than 50,000 Units, B.P., 10,000 Units, U.S.P.

Scarlet Fever Antitoxin, B.P., is similarly prepared from an animal immunized against the toxin produced by the streptococcus regarded as causative of scarlet fever.

Gas-gangrene Antitoxins. The B.P. contains three different antitoxins to combat gas-gangrene according to the type of organism producing the condition, viz. *Gas-gangrene Antitoxin (Oedematiens)*, *(Septicum)*, and *(Welchii)*, and *Mixed Gas-Gangrene Antitoxin*, containing all three.

The presence of antibacterial and antitoxic substances in the blood of persons who have recovered from a variety of diseases confers lasting immunity on these individuals but it is seldom possible to make practical use of this source of antibodies in the protection of those exposed to infection. There is available in the U.S.P. *Pertussis Immune Human Serum* which is the liquid or dried serum of a healthy person who has recovered recently from whooping-cough. Three or four injections of 20 ml. intramuscularly may abort the more serious symptoms of pertussis in an infant.

In addition infants may be entirely protected from measles, or a mild attack of this ubiquitous disease may be permitted by giving an appropriate dose of *Immune Serum Globulin*, U.S.P. This is a sterile preparation of the globulin fraction of human serum which contains most of the antibodies in the blood. It is prepared from a pooled source of not less than one thousand individuals. A similar preparation of immune globulin may be used to attenuate attacks of poliomyelitis. It is to be noted that these products do not come from individual donors who have recently survived an attack of the disease, but from a common pool. This is possible because the antibodies are found in the majority of adult bloods. They are concentrated (globulin fraction) and they are tested for potency before use.

B. ACTIVE IMMUNIZATION

I. VACCINES

As has already been pointed out, natural cure of bacterial diseases results largely from the formation in the blood and tissues of 'antibodies' which prevent the multiplication of bacteria or neutralize their toxins. Immunity acquired in this way—whereby the person infected manufactures his own antibodies as the result of an attack of the disease—is called 'Active Immunity', as contrasted to the 'Passive Immunity' which is conferred by injection of an antitoxin or antibacterial serum obtained from an immunized animal. Active immunity is usually more complete and permanent than passive immunity, but can only be gained by undergoing the disease. A mild attack of a disease may confer almost as complete immunity as a severe attack. In the case of some diseases it would be worth while, therefore, to undergo a mild attack in order to be immunized against the possibility of a severe or even fatal attack. This is virtually what is done in vaccination against smallpox. One drop of vaccine lymph, *Smallpox Vaccine*, B.P., U.S.P. (which is obtained from the vesicles produced by inoculation of vaccinia virus on the skin of healthy animals), is applied by scarification or pressure inoculation to the skin of the human patient. This provokes a reaction resembling in some ways a mild attack of smallpox and which suffices to confer a partial or absolute immunity against smallpox, lasting many years.

It has been found that injected bacteria, even when they are killed, can often provoke active immunity, so that a person can be immunized to such bacteria with relatively little risk, because the bacteria cannot multiply in the body. Advantage of this fact is taken in vaccination against typhoid fevers. It has already been pointed out that antibodies are highly specific and act only upon the particular toxin or bacterium that has provoked their formation. There are four bacilli, viz. *Salmonella typhi*, and *Salmonella paratyphi A, B*, and *C*, which are responsible for different kinds of typhoid fever. Though they are closely allied, an attack due to infection by one of these bacilli will not confer immunity to the others. In order to immunize a person simultaneously to the three principal organisms, it is now the practice to use a vaccine containing all three, e.g. *Typhoid and Paratyphoid A and B Vaccine*, B.P., (T.A.B. Vaccine), *Typhoid-Paratyphoid Vaccine*, U.S.P. This is a standardized sterile suspension of those three bacilli which have been killed by heating. Two doses can be given by subcutaneous injection, the first of 0·5 ml. and the second, 7 days later, of 1·0 ml. Such vaccination has been practised on a large scale and has greatly lowered the incidence and severity of typhoid fevers.

There are also available a *Typhoid-Paratyphoid A, B, and C, Vaccine*, B.P. (T.A.B.C. Vaccine), which includes all four species of Salmonella, and a Typhoid-Paratyphoid Vaccine with Tetanus Toxoid which performs a double function.

If the disease is known to be due to the *S. typhi* proper, the necessity for a mixed vaccine does not arise, and a simple vaccine (*Typhoid Vaccine*, U.S.P.) can be used.

Vaccination against smallpox or typhoid fevers is, of course, a prophylactic vaccination. Vaccines have been employed similarly against a variety of infectious diseases. *Vaccines* which are common to the B.P. and U.S.P. include those against *Cholera, Plague, Epidemic Typhus*, and *Yellow Fever*. The U.S.P. also includes a *Rabies Vaccine*. In order to induce an effective degree of active immunity, these vaccines have usually, as with typhoid vaccine, to be administered on at least two occasions, separated as a rule by an interval of 7–10 days or more.

Whooping-Cough Vaccine, B.P., is a specially prepared starch suspension of *Haemophilus pertussis*, given for the prophylaxis of whooping-cough in three doses of 20,000 million bacilli at intervals of 4 weeks. An *Alum Precipitated Pertussis Vaccine* is official in the U.S.P.

Bacillus Calmette-Guerin Vaccine, B.P., confers a degree of immunity on those who are adjudged by preliminary testing with tuberculin (p. 262) to be susceptible to tuberculosis. This, like smallpox vaccine, is prepared from a strain of living but attenuated organisms.

II. TOXINS AND TOXOIDS

The pathological effects produced by bacterial infections are in many cases due chiefly to toxins formed by the bacteria. These toxins can often be separated from the bacteria in a moderately pure state. They may be obtained, for example, in the filtrate from the culture of the bacteria grown in a fluid medium.

In many diseases it is preferable to immunize against the toxin rather than against the bacterium itself, and just as immunity can often be provoked by injection of devitalized bacteria, so immunity can also be provoked by injection of attenuated toxins. Various methods have been tried for reducing the virulence of a toxin without destroying its power of provoking immunity. This can sometimes be done successfully by addition to the toxin of the specific antitoxin or of formaldehyde, or by precipitation with alum. Such procedures are adopted in the case of *Diphtheria Prophylactic*, B.P., *Diphtheria Toxoid*, U.S.P. Active immunity which may last for years can be induced in children by injecting small doses of the toxoid. In the B.P. *Diphtheria Prophylactic* is permissible in the following forms: (*a*) *Formol Toxoid* (F.T.), (*b*) *Alum Precipitated Toxoid* (A.P.T.), (*c*) *Purified Toxoid, Aluminium Phosphate* (P.T.A.P.), and (*d*) *Toxoid-Antitoxin Floccules* (T.A.F.). In the U.S.P. there are *Diphtheria Toxoid* (which is treated with formaldehyde), *Alum Precipitated Diphtheria Toxoid*, and *Diphtheria Toxoid, Aluminum Hydroxide Adsorbed*.

Some people have a high natural resistance to diphtheria, and it is not so necessary to immunize these. The susceptibility to diphtheria can be gauged by the Schick Test. This consists in the intradermal injection of a minute amount of specially prepared toxin. Persons who are sensitive to diphtheria develop an area of redness at the site of injection. For thus diagnosing the existence of a predisposition to diphtheria, *Schick Test Toxin*, B.P., *Diagnostic Diphtheria Toxin*, U.S.P., is used (0·2 ml. by intradermal injection). A positive reaction (i.e. redness at the site of injection) is not proof positive of sensitiveness to diphtheria, for in some people such an effect may result as a reaction not to the toxin itself but to non-specific substances contained in the so-called toxin, which is not pure toxin. In order to exclude this possibility a control test is done in this way. An intradermal injection of the same amount is given simultaneously into the opposite arm of the same diagnostic toxin, which has been previously heated so as to destroy the toxin. The toxin so heated is called *Schick Control*, B.P., *Inactivated Diagnostic Diphtheria Toxin*, U.S.P.

A complete positive reaction, indicating a susceptible individual, is shown by an area of redness at the site of injection of the diagnostic toxin but no such area at the site of injection of the heated toxin. Persons showing this complete positive reaction of susceptibility can then with advantage be actively immunized by injections of Diptheria Prophylactic as already explained.

In connexion with the disease diphtheria, the B.P. therefore contains three quite distinct preparations: (1) Schick Test Toxin, which, together with Schick Control, is used especially in the *diagnosis* of susceptibility to diphtheria; (2) Diphtheria Prophylactic, which is used to induce active immunity in susceptible persons, and is therefore chiefly concerned with the *prophylaxis* of diphtheria; (3) Diphtheria Antitoxin, which contains the antibodies formed by an artificially immunized animal, and is used chiefly in the *treatment* of diphtheria, to confer a passive immunity.

Another toxoid (the name 'toxoid' merely indicates that the activity of the toxin has been artificially reduced) used for inducing active immunity is tetanus toxoid. Fortunately, tetanus is a disease not so prevalent among the general population as to necessitate mass inoculation against it, and tetanus toxoid is used chiefly in the prophylactic active immunization of soldiers on active service. *Tetanus Toxoid* may be used in simple solution or in *Alum Precipitated* form, B.P., U.S.P., or as *Aluminum Hydroxide Adsorbed Tetanus Toxoid*, U.S.P.

Staphylococcus Toxoid, B.P., contains a sterile diluted toxoid of a pathogenic strain of *Staphyloccocus*, which may be of value in the treatment of chronic furunculosis.

Mention was made of the skin test for possible susceptibility to tuberculosis. For this purpose a concentrated filtrate from a fluid medium on which has grown a suitable strain of *Mycobacterium tuberculosis* may be used—*Old Tuberculin*, B.P., or perhaps preferably the *Purified Protein Derivative of Tuberculin*, B.P., U.S.P., which is prepared by fractional precipitation and subsequent freeze-drying of the above. It is less likely to give false readings due to non-specific allergens.

ANAPHYLAXIS

Before leaving the subject of immunization, reference must be made to the condition of anaphylaxis which appears superficially to be the opposite of immunity, though it is in fact merely an incidental possibility in the immunization process. When an antigen is injected into an animal, it provokes the formation of antibodies in the blood which precipitate the antigen and render it inert. If a small dose of antigen is injected, the antibodies circulate in the blood for a few days and after a week or so are found mostly in the tissues. If, when this occurs, a second injection of antigen is given and there is not sufficient antibody in the blood to combine with it, the antigen combines with the antibodies in the tissues and the consequent precipitation inside the cell may provoke a reaction called anaphylaxis. The resulting symptoms, being partly due to release of histamine, (p. 180), will depend upon the cells affected, but they are manifested especially in smooth muscle and most conspicuously in that of the bronchi, constriction of which causes an acute attack of asthma. Less commonly, nausea, vomiting, or diarrhoea may occur. Anaphylaxis may occur to any protein and is highly specific to the particular protein used. In practice it may occur with antitoxic sera but the development of more highly purified sera together with the recognition of the importance of judicious dosage and timing has much diminished the frequency of its occurrence. In specially sensitive persons or with large intravenous doses of serum (which should never be given to asthmatics) the danger is still present.

An anaphylactic reaction may appear within a few minutes up to 2 hours after an injection. Another allied type of reaction, called serum sickness, may occur after several days, often about a week. Among the symptoms are fever, pains in the muscles and joints, and skin rashes, especially urticarial, which may cause intense irritation.

The immediate treatment for all anaphylactic symptoms is an intramuscular injection of adrenaline, followed if necessary by ephedrine orally.

Anaphylaxis as described above may be regarded as acquired anaphylaxis, but some persons have an inborn sensitiveness to certain proteins and may, for example, show similar symptoms as the result of a first injection of serum. Inhalation of many proteins, e.g. in pollen, moulds, horse and cat dandruff, or ingestion of certain foodstuffs may in hypersensitive persons produce allergic reactions allied to anaphylaxis, especially asthma, hay-fever, eczema, and other skin rashes. This predisposition is frequently hereditary. If a particular protein is proved to be responsible, it may be possible to desensitize the patient to it by giving repeated small doses. Allergic effects are not confined to proteins but occur with many drugs. Aspirin in a small proportion of people may produce asthma or urticaria.

XXIII

CHEMOTHERAPY

PROTOZOAL organisms are responsible for many widespread and important diseases, and in these diseases antitoxins or vaccines have proved of little therapeutic or prophylactic value as compared with chemical agents. Indeed the failure of antitoxic treatment in protozoal diseases was one factor which stimulated the search for chemical remedies. Treatment by these remedies is often called *Chemotherapy*, a word originally employed to differentiate therapy by means of chemical agents, often synthetic and of which the composition was known, from therapy by means of antitoxins, which, though no doubt also chemical entities, had not been isolated, could not be artificially manufactured, and the exact composition of which was unknown.

Chemotherapy, e.g. the use of quinine in malaria or of mercury in syphilis, goes back centuries; but the few known remedies of this inheritance, though important, had been discovered by the empiric use of drugs in diseases in man, a slow and uncertain process of investigation by which little advance had been made. A new impetus to the subject was given by Ehrlich's investigations into the chemotherapy of experimental trypanosomiasis (p. 292), because they established the possibility of discovering new and important remedies by means of experiments on laboratory animals. He used small animals, e.g. mice, which are susceptible to certain trypanosome infections, and which, when so infected, can be used to test the remedial value of a potential remedy. Thus not only the symptomatology and toxicity (pharmacology) of a chemical compound, but also its efficacy in a disease (therapeutics) could be determined in a single species of animal. The use of small laboratory animals, apart from any humane reasons, greatly facilitated investigation, for a large number of animals could be used with limited accommodation and at low cost. Moreover, a disease like trypanosomiasis runs a shorter course in a small animal than in man, corresponding to the shorter life of the animal itself. Results can therefore be obtained in a much shorter time, and, in the artificially induced disease, the exact type and degree of the infection are under control.

For this type of investigation two factors are necessary, the possibility of communicating an infection to laboratory animals, and the discovery of a chemical compound which has some remedial action in the infection. With regard to the first factor, the discovery of new therapeutic agents has run roughly parallel with the ease of inducing a particular infection in small animals. With regard to the second factor, once a compound of known chemical composition is discovered which has some remedial action in the disease, new related compounds can be synthesized with the object of finding one which will have a lower toxicity for the host and a higher toxicity for the pathogenic organism, so as to obtain a more potent remedy possessing a greater margin of safety in use.

By these methods and with these experimental advantages, chemotherapeutic investigations are being vigorously conducted with a view to discovering remedies against almost every known type of infection. Success at first was attained mainly in the realm of protozoal maladies, but more recently and, especially with the sulphonamides, penicillin, and other antibiotics, remarkable progress has been made in the discovery of remedies against bacterial infections. It is an understatement to say that more progress in practical therapeutics has been made by modern chemotherapeutic methods of investigation in a decade than could be made in a century by the empirical trial of natural remedies in naturally occurring disease.

It may be instructive here to glance back at some of the *landmarks in the progress of chemotherapy*.

In 1907 Ehrlich introduced arsphenamine (p. 73), an organic compound of arsenic, for the treatment of syphilis and allied diseases. The practical success of his ideas and experimental methods stimulated further researches on arsenical compounds which led to the introduction of new and improved remedies for diseases of this type. In 1921 bismuth (p. 68), as a result of preliminary laboratory research, was introduced clinically for the treatment of syphilis and soon almost completely replaced mercury which had been used for centuries as a remedy for this disease. Later antimony (p. 69) was found also to have a trypanocidal action and proved a successful remedy for another group of protozoal diseases—leishmaniasis. Within a quarter of a century of Ehrlich's discovery of salvarsan, chemotherapy had achieved remarkable successes which had completely altered the outlook of many of the most important diseases.

There was, however, one discouraging aspect. The progress was almost confined to diseases due to protozoa. The older chemical agents which had been discovered empirically and which had proved successful remedies—mercury in syphilis, quinine in malaria, and ipecacuanha in amoebic dysentery—were also restricted to protozoal diseases. Chemotherapy had as yet made no worth-while contribution to the treatment of that large number of important diseases due to bacterial or virus infections. It almost seemed as if chemical agents were to be of no avail in the attack upon these diseases, in which case reliance would have to be placed upon treatment by antitoxins.

In 1935 these doubts were dispelled by the introduction of the sulphonamide group of drugs (p. 272), some of which proved superior to any hitherto known remedies for bacterial infections. Apart from the immediate therapeutic gain, this was of fundamental importance because it showed conclusively that pathogenic bacteria, as well as pathogenic protozoa, were susceptible to chemotherapy.

An even more dramatic discovery was in the offing. In 1929 Fleming had discovered the remarkable bacteriostatic properties of penicillin (p. 281), a substance released by a mould in the culture medium in which it grew. From 1940 onwards this discovery was developed to a practical conclusion by Florey, Chain, and their colleagues. Penicillin was found to have a unique range of therapeutic activity, being active against many diseases, pneumonia, gonorrhoea, syphilis, &c. Not only so, but this advance opened up a whole new field of chemotherapy —by substances derived from various fungi, bacteria, &c., sometimes grouped under the inclusive name of 'antibiotics'. True, there were still pathogenic organisms which were scarcely affected by either sulphonamides or penicillin. That inveterate and indomitable enemy of mankind, the tubercle bacillus, was one. Further exploration of antibiotics, however, revealed one substance, streptomycin, which is of value in tuberculous infections, against which hitherto no remedy had been of any avail. More recently, simpler synthetic compounds have been discovered which are of curative value in these infections.

The advances have been on a broad front. New and effective chemotherapeutic remedies have been discovered for such scourges as pneumonia, malaria, venereal diseases, typhoid and typhus fevers, anthrax, leprosy, plague, and many others. Progress, slower and more difficult, is being made with virus infections.

In face of these brilliant and fruitful discoveries which have caused a revolution in medical treatment and outlook it may seem grudging to issue a warning against the too optimistic view that all is over except the shouting. Not only pathogenic microorganisms but also the insect vectors of disease have shown a subtle resistance to most chemotherapeutic remedies, especially if they are given time. A long view reveals many unsolved problems and some cause for solicitude. Some factors in this reaction of micro-organisms will be discussed in the next section.

DRUG TOLERANCE ACQUIRED BY MICRO-ORGANISMS

To man's intensified chemotherapeutic attack upon their parasitic vested rights, pathogenic micro-organisms are not without their means of defence. Unicellular organisms could hardly have persisted for millions of years since the dawn of life without possessing boundless resource and adaptability. One of these means must be mentioned, as it is of fundamental and far-reaching importance for chemotherapy generally.

In the course of his original experiments with atoxyl (p. 73), Ehrlich found that, when a mouse was infected with trypanosomes, an injection of atoxyl might cause partial or complete disappearance of trypanosomes from the blood. If the trypanosomes had all been killed the animal was cured. More often, however (owing to the difficulty of giving a sufficient dose to kill all the trypanosomes without killing the mouse itself), trypanosomes multiplied again in the blood after an interval. If the mouse now received a second injection of the same dose of atoxyl this had less effect than the first, as shown by the facts that more trypanosomes survived the injection and multiplication occurred after a shorter interval. Repeated injections of atoxyl became progressively less effective in killing the trypanosomes. If now a second mouse was infected with these resistant trypanosomes, they were still equally insensitive to atoxyl and they, in fact, retained this property even after repeated transmissions from mouse to mouse, until finally a stage might be reached when the trypanosomes were totally unaffected even by many times that dose of atoxyl that originally would have caused complete disappearance of trypanosomes from the blood. An atoxyl-resistant 'strain' of trypanosomes had emerged as the result of treatment and, as they multiply by simple fission, this property was preserved for generations—possibly in perpetuity. Subsequent experience has revealed that this facility for acquiring resistance is possessed more or less by most, if not all, micro-organisms, bacteria as well as trypanosomes, and applies to a greater or less degree to most chemotherapeutic agents.

This first became obvious in the treatment of gonorrhoea with sulphonamides. At first so successful, they were soon found to be more and more frequently ineffectual. Gonococci isolated from those cases were found to be sulphonamide-resistant and cases infected with such a strain failed to respond to sulphonamide treatment. That the acquisition of resistance is not universal is shown by the facts that the meningococcus, so closely related biochemically to the gonococcus, develops little resistance to sulphonamides and that the gonococcus so far shows little sign of developing serious resistance to penicillin.

The risk attending the production of resistant strains of pathogenic organisms is of practical importance in the treatment of diseases, especially in two ways. In the first place it may influence the continuing efficacy of a drug in an individual patient, especially if repeated doses have to be given over a period and if the drug used is one to which micro-organisms rapidly acquire tolerance. For example, if a case of tuberculous meningitis is treated with streptomycin (p. 284), the bacilli may acquire a high degree of resistance to it in a few days and, should the disease not be cured or should there be a relapse, later treatment with streptomycin may be wholly ineffective.

In the second place a resistant strain of micro-organisms may affect the treatment of populations. To take an extreme example, in certain districts of Africa where trypanosomiasis is prevalent and nearly all cases have been treated with an arsenical compound without stamping out the disease, arsenical compounds have almost entirely lost their therapeutic efficacy because the disease is now being maintained by a strain of trypanosomes resistant to arsenic.

How micro-organisms acquire such resistance is not yet certain. Undoubtedly one factor is survival of the fittest. In a population of organisms, some individuals are from the beginning more resistant than others, e.g. may survive several times the concentration of a drug that will kill the majority of their fellows. The non-resistant individuals may be killed but those resistant survive and multiply. Whether an individual organism can, when subjected to the action of a drug, acquire in its own lifetime a transmissible tolerance, is not so certain.

Almost certainly resistance may be due in some cases to the emergence of drug-resistant mutants selected in the presence of a drug. An organism may acquire resistance to penicillin by developing a penicillinase which destroys the antibiotic before it can affect the organism. Clearly micro-organisms can acquire resistance in different ways and much has to be done before the factors can be elucidated.

How far this problem is likely to affect chemotherapy in the more distant future it is too early to say. Certainly as time goes on more organisms are acquiring resistance to more antibiotics, which may then become therapeutically useless. New substances can replace them for a time. Though generally resistance is specific for a particular drug, cross tolerance may occur if two compounds are nearly related, e.g. aureomycin and terramycin, so that organisms which have developed resistance to one are found to be also resistant to the other.

Some disconcerting results have followed the use of antibiotics in mixed infections. If an antibiotic kills off one sensitive species of bacterium, another insensitive or resistant species may flourish. For example, in some hospitals the staphylococcus has almost entirely replaced the haemolytic streptococcus as a cause of epidemic hospital sepsis. One explanation (others are possible) is that streptococci do not easily acquire resistance to antibiotics whereas staphylococci unfortunately do. With the general and extensive use of antibiotics the streptococci are killed off, leaving the ground clear for drug-resistant staphylococci.

Fortunately there are some factors on the credit side. To some drugs organisms can develop little resistance, e.g. much less to mercury than to arsenic; and this may explain why mercury did not lose its efficacy against syphilis even after centuries of use. Treatment by a combination or alternation of different chemotherapeutic agents may retard or prevent the development of resistance to any one of them. In the treatment of tuberculosis, p-aminosalicylic acid or isoniazid or both together, given along with streptomycin not only have a summative curative effect but also delay the development of streptomycin-resistance in the bacillus.

The practical lesson is plain: (1) it is important to endeavour to cure an individual patient by sufficient doses and as quickly as possible before the pathogenic organism acquires resistance to the drug; (2) it is important to prevent the spread of an infection transmitted by organisms which have already acquired resistance; (3) the widespread and indiscriminate use of antibiotics, especially for minor maladies or in ineffective doses must be discouraged. Otherwise they may fail in cases where they might have been life-saving. If a drug has a unique action in some serious disease, it should be withheld in other diseases for which an alternative antibiotic is available.

XXIV

DRUGS USED IN BACTERIAL INFECTIONS

SYSTEMIC ANTISEPTICS

SOME problems involved in the local use of antiseptics have been considered in Chapter XXII, together with some of the drugs which are in common use for this purpose.

The problem is more difficult and the choice of antiseptic more limited when the attempt is made to inhibit bacterial growth in distal organs or whenever the antiseptic has to be conveyed by the blood stream. All the organs in the body are exposed to the action of an antiseptic in the blood, and it is difficult to find a substance which will inhibit bacterial growth in a concentration which will be innocuous, especially to the more delicate organs of the body.

SULPHONAMIDES

In the last few years a more hopeful outlook on the treatment of streptococcal and other infections has been brought about as the result of the discovery of new chemotherapeutic agents. This began with the discovery by Domagk in 1935 that a substance called Prontosil rubrum had a pronounced action in preventing and curing infections with haemolytic streptococci. This is a red dye only slightly soluble in water, given by oral administration. Later soluble compounds were introduced suitable for parenteral administration, e.g. prontosil soluble, soluseptasine. It was found that, after administration of prontosil, large amounts of a simpler compound, *p*-aminobenzenesulphonamide, were excreted in the urine and the activity of prontosil compounds was believed to be due to the liberation of this substance, which then came to be used by itself under various names, of which the name Sulphanilamide is now official.

Subsequently some hundreds of derivatives of sulphanilamide have been synthesized and biologically tested with the aim
of discovering drugs superior to sulphanilamide for the treatment of various infections. The composition of some of the
most important of these is given in the following Table.

Constitution of some Sulphonamides and of Dapsone

*In the 2nd to 4th compounds the terminal —H of Sulphanilamide
is replaced by the group indicated*

Sulphanilamide	NH_2⟨ ⟩$SO_2 \cdot N \cdot$ $\overset{\text{H}}{\underset{}{	}}$—H
Sulphacetamide Sodium	—$NaCO \cdot CH_3$
Sulphadiazine	—$C\overset{N—CH}{\underset{N=CH}{\diagdown}}CH$
Sulphaguanidine	—$C\overset{NH_2}{\underset{NH}{\diagdown}}$
Dapsone	H_2N⟨ ⟩SO_2⟨ ⟩NH_2

These compounds differ considerably from one another in
their relative bactericidal actions on different types of bacteria
and also in their physical properties which influence their absorption, excretion, and concentration in the blood. Consequently it has been found that one compound may be more
effective than another in the treatment of a particular disease.
There are, however, certain properties common to this group
of drugs which may be mentioned first. When a compound is
given with a view to its absorption, the therapeutic result depends upon the effective concentration in the blood. Especially
in *acute* infections it is important to begin with a large initial
dose so as to raise the blood concentration of the drug as quickly
as possible; in very severe cases the first dose may be given
parenterally. The advantage of getting the blood concentration

high to begin with is that the drug acts more effectively the fewer the number of organisms and, therefore, before they have had time to multiply; also the organisms may acquire some degree of tolerance to the drug if it is administered repeatedly in too small doses. The concentration of the compound in the blood should be kept at an effective level throughout the whole day, especially in the acute stages of an infection. This usually necessitates giving the drug orally every four hours, day and night, for a few days. The dosage is reduced as the condition improves. As a rule, sulphonamide treatment should be continued for two or three days after the patient's temperature has become normal, and the total duration of treatment should seldom exceed a week. In regard to actual doses, it is impossible to give a brief statement that might not be misleading, as dosage naturally depends upon the stage and severity of the disease, the age of the patient, and the tolerance exhibited to the drug. Generally, however, the *dosage* in a severe infection may be of the order of 3 G. as an initial dose, followed by 1 G. 4-hourly for two or three days, after which this dose can be given less frequently.

Part of the absorbed sulphonamide is acetylated in the liver to a degree varying with different compounds and probably with different individuals. The acetyl derivative is usually less soluble than the parent compound. In the course of excretion by the kidney, the concentration of the drug may be raised, e.g. from 2 mg. per 100 ml. in the blood to 100 mg. per 100 ml. in the urine. At this increased concentration, the acetyl derivative may be incompletely soluble and, in the case of the less soluble sulphonamides, be precipitated as crystals in the renal tubes or ureters, giving rise to lumbar pain, haematuria, or even anuria. The risk of this occurrence can be lessened by administering a large fluid intake and also by simultaneous administration of alkalis which increase the solubility in the urine. When these particular compounds are given, regular watch must be kept for the occurrence of lumbar pain, diminution of urinary output, and haematuria, which may necessitate reduction in dosage of the drug or even its discontinuance.

It could hardly be expected that drugs of this degree of potency should be entirely free from undesirable actions, especially if the single or total dosage is high. Among the toxic actions which have been described, in addition to those mentioned involving the urinary excretion, are nausea and vomiting; cyanosis due to formation of methaemoglobin or sulphaemoglobin; mental confusion or depression; drug fever and skin rashes; leucopenia or, in rare cases, agranulocytosis; acute haemolytic anaemia. The more serious of these effects are rare.

In general sulphonamides are not a success when applied locally as crystals, ointments, or creams and there is a grave danger of the patient developing local or general reactions such as hypersensitivity to light. With the exception of *Sulphacetamide Sodium*, B.P., U.S.P., which may be used as an *Eye Ointment* (6 per cent. B.P., 10 per cent. U.S.P.), topical application is to be avoided.

Sulphonamides are not effective against viruses, tubercle, enterococci, anaerobes, or in rheumatism, but are of value in the treatment of infections due to many common Gram-positive organisms. In one infection, meningococcal meningitis, sulphadiazine or sulphamerazine is the drug of choice.

The mode of action of sulphonamide is by competition with factors essential to bacterial growth, such as p-aminobenzoic acid and folinic acid (p. 234), for limited enzyme available in the bacterium. The object of treatment is to produce a sufficient concentration of sulphonamide at the site of infection to have a bacteriostatic effect, i.e. to prevent further increase in numbers of bacteria.

The attributes and uses of individual compounds may now be briefly mentioned. The first eight compounds are all official in the B.P. or U.S.P.

Sulphanilamide, B.P., is the simplest, cheapest, and most easily synthesized of the compounds mentioned and is effective especially in haemolytic streptococcal infections, e.g. cellulitis, erysipelas, puerperal sepsis, &c. Cyanosis, usually not of serious import, is common with this compound, but depression occurs rarely, and the kidney seems not to be affected owing to the high solubility of acetyl-sulphanilamide. It commonly gives rise to nausea and vomiting, and with the introduction of less toxic and equally effective compounds its use is now largely abandoned.

Sulphathiazole, B.P., has a wide range of therapeutic uses. It has been found especially effective in staphylococcal, pneumococcal, meningococcal, and gonococcal infections. Other serious toxic effects occur rarely with it, but the urinary secretion must be watched as the acetyl derivative is relatively insoluble. For this reason its popularity is limited unless in mixture with other sulphonamides.

Sulphadiazine, B.P., U.S.P., is used in much the same conditions as sulphathiazole, which it closely resembles in effects. It is usually well tolerated, rarely causes vomiting, and is relatively free from undesirable actions, apart from the possibility of kidney trouble. The sodium salt of this sulphonamide is of value for intravenous administration.

Sulfamerazine, U.S.P., is another pyrimidine derivative which differs from sulphadiazine only in the methylation of one carbon in the substituent ring, whereas in its congener *Sulphadimidine*, B.P., *Sulfamethazine*, U.S.P., two methyl groups have been added. These changes have produced compounds which are more rapidly absorbed and more slowly excreted than sulphadiazine. They therefore offer the great advantage that dosage need not be so frequent and that adequate blood and tissue levels of the drug are more easily maintained overnight. As absorption is also less complete the initial dose may be raised to 3–4 G. and the maintenance dose of 1 G. given at 6–8-hour intervals. The solubility in urine is good. The sodium salts may be administered intravenously in case of necessity and have the advantage of penetrating to the cerebrospinal fluid to a degree which is superior to that of most sulphonamides. They are thus preferred for the treatment of meningococcal meningitis. Sulphadimidine is probably the most frequently prescribed of all sulphonamides for routine purposes.

Absorption of the above compounds is usually sufficiently rapid and complete from the alimentary canal. Exceptionally in diseases with high mortality rates (e.g. meningitis) or in unconscious patients, some sulphonamides may be injected parenterally. The normal compounds, with the exception of sulphanilamide, are too insoluble, but the official *Sodium* salts of *Sulphathiazole* and *Sulphadimidine*, B.P., *Sulfadiazine*, and *Sulfamerazine*, U.S.P., are freely soluble. Mainly owing to their high alkalinity, solutions of these salts are too irritating for subcutaneous injection. Even intramuscular injection may cause local sloughing. They are therefore given intravenously and they must be sterile. They are injected slowly in 5–10 per cent. solution.

Sulphacetamide Sodium, B.P., U.S.P., is the salt of N-sulphanilyl acetamide, i.e. it must be differentiated from the acetyl derivatives of sulphonamides which are the relatively insoluble products in which the acetylation occurs on the para-amino group, the opposite end of the molecule. It is extremely soluble, not as alkaline as the sodium salts of other sulphonamides, and therefore of use in such conditions as inflammation of the eyelids (p. 275). The parent body may be used as a systemic sulphonamide. It is well absorbed.

In contrast to the foregoing compounds, the next three owe their particular sphere of use to the fact that they are relatively very feebly absorbed from the alimentary canal.

Sulphaguanidine, B.P., though readily soluble, is very imperfectly absorbed from the alimentary canal and most of it remains in the intestine and is excreted in the faeces. As it is active against certain intestinal bacteria, it thus has the full opportunity of developing its action on them, without enough being absorbed to produce systemic toxic actions. It has been used especially in bacillary dysentery. It has no beneficial effect in typhoid fevers. Dosage is relatively high, 3–6 G.

Succinylsulphathiazole, B.P., dose 3–6 G., U.S.P., dose 2 Gm. 4-hourly, is also only slightly absorbed from the alimentary canal and can be given without causing toxic symptoms in bacillary infections of the intestine.

Phthalylsulfathiazole, U.S.P., has similar properties and uses to succinylsulphathiazole.

Sulfisoxazole, U.S.P., (Sulphafurazole), may be given in

initial doses of 4 Gm. for the treatment of infections of the urinary tract, especially with *Proteus* organisms. where no mechanical obstruction exists to the free flow of urine. It is readily absorbed, very soluble, and therefore not likely to deposit urinary crystals when present in high concentration in the urine.

SULPHONES AND LEPROSY

Hydnocarpus Oil, B.P., and chaulmoogra oil were long used as a remedy for leprosy. The oils were taken by mouth but caused so much gastric irritation that effective doses could not be given. Preparations such as **Injection of Hydnocarpus Oil**, B.P., or **Injection of Ethyl Esters of Hydnocarpus Oil**, B.P., 2–5 ml., were given with greater success, but of recent years they have been almost abandoned owing to the vastly superior results obtained with the following sulphone compounds.

Dapsone (diamino-diphenyl-sulphone) is reminiscent of a sulphonamide but the essential structural difference should be noted. It is a symmetrical sulphone. Given by mouth in doses of 0·1–0·3 G. per day in long courses it brings about remarkable improvement in lepromatous and tuberculoid infections due to the leprosy bacillus. Readily absorbed, it tends to give rise to high tissue concentrations, and toxic side-effects are rather common. They may take the form of reactions of the skin or the eyes, apart from temporary illness due to the sudden release of leprous toxins from the killed bacilli. These reactions, though giving evidence of therapeutic success, may be severe.

The U.S.P. contains **Sulfoxone Sodium**, dose 300 mg. daily, in which the amino groups are methylated, and the propyl-amino analogue Solapsone is also in use. The further substitution makes absorption take place more slowly and thus avoids many of the toxic effects encountered with Dapsone.

ANTIBIOTICS

Antibiotics have been defined by Waksman, who introduced the word in 1942, as 'chemical substances that are produced by micro-organisms and that have the capacity, in dilute solution, to inhibit the growth, and even to destroy, other micro-organisms'. The role of these substances in nature is presumably to act as exotoxins which discourage the growth and reproduction of competitors for the nutrient media which harbour primitive forms of life.

Antibiotics are produced by various groups of micro-organisms, especially (*a*) *Bacillus* and *Pseudomonas*, which mostly produce polypeptides, e.g. tyrothricin and polymixin; (*b*) fungi, only one important group, the penicillins; (*c*) *Actinomyces*, e.g. streptomycin, chloramphenicol, tetracycline. During the last fifteen years several hundred antibiotics have been isolated; only about a score have found a place as chemotherapeutic agents.

Antibiotics vary greatly in chemical composition. Some contain C, H, and O, e.g. clavicin; some C, H, O, and N, e.g. streptomycin; some C, H, O, N, and S, e.g. penicillin; some C, H, O, N, with Cl, e.g. chloramphenicol. The precise structure of a few of them is known but only one, chloramphenicol, is regularly synthesized. The others are obtained from the liquors in which cultures of the appropriate fungi or bacteria are grown. Special media and conditions of cultivation are necessary for their production.

Antibiotics vary greatly in their selective action on different micro-organisms. The range of this selective action is often referred to as the 'spectrum' of the antibiotic. Some act on bacteria, some on fungi, some on the larger viruses, and some on protozoa; others have combinations of these actions. With this wide range of activity antibiotics have found extensive use in the treatment of a great variety of diseases in men and animals. It is not an overstatement to say that they have revolutionized the treatment and prognosis of many of the most widespread and serious diseases. They are also used in plant diseases, animal feeding, and in preservation of biological materials.

The mode of action of antibiotics is but little understood but in the case of penicillin and streptomycin these antibiotics are much more effective against actively growing and dividing bacteria than against resting ones. Penicillin would appear to inhibit enzymes which catalyse synthesis of certain essential amino-acids, to inhibit utilization of glutamic acid compounds, and to interfere with the metabolism of ribonucleic acid. The mode of action of streptomycin is different, being concerned with a phase of oxygen utilization. Many antibiotics are only bactericidal in concentrations which harm tissue cells, many are not bactericidal even in high concentration, whereas with tyrothricin, for instance, doubling the concentration changes the action from inhibition of bacterial growth to sterilization. Selection and proper use of the most effective antibiotic for any given infection is important because of two factors: (a) the differing 'antibacterial spectra' of the individual antibiotics, which makes it necessary to be sure that the agent used is capable of affecting the organism concerned. Mixtures of antibiotics may be used for topical application to infections which have not been cultured; (b) the development of resistance in bacteria (p. 267). This phenomenon is particularly encountered with *Staphylococcus* in relation to penicillin and with *Mycobacterium* in relation to streptomycin. The therapeutic usefulness of penicillin in relation to staphyloccocal infection is threatened by this phenomenon, and that of streptomycin would be very limited indeed were it not for the use of other substances in conjunction with the antibiotic.

All antibiotics produce toxic symptoms in some people. Penicillin sensitivity takes the form of an urticarial rash which may be controlled with antihistamines, but occasionally a dangerous anaphylactic collapse has occurred. Streptomycin has its special selective toxicity on the eighth nerve and, like penicilin, may give much trouble to nursing staff from contact dermatitis. The orally administered antibiotics often cause diarrhoea or vomiting and all of them may give rise to acute vitamin deficiencies by suppression of the normal intestinal bacterial flora which synthesizes certain elements of the B complex. Another complication which has resulted from the absence of normal flora is the growth of yeasts and fungi. Thrush and similar infections may spread rapidly in the mouth, intestine, vagina, &c.

It may therefore be concluded that antibiotics, while they are of supreme importance as antimicrobial agents, must be used with discrimination and skill if the best results are to be obtained.

PENICILLIN

In 1929 Alexander Fleming noticed that when a mould—*Penicillium notatum*—grew on a culture plate along with staphylococci, the latter underwent lysis in an area surrounding the mould. He found that the mould had liberated into the culture medium a bactericidal substance which he called penicillin. He showed that the action of this substance was specific for certain organisms and that it had a very low toxicity. About a decade later, Florey, Chain, and their colleagues proceeded to purify extracts of penicillin and to determine their bactericidal activity *in vitro* and *in vivo*, including as many experiments on man as their limited amount of material allowed. Stimulated by the success of their results, the manufacture of penicillin was launched on a large scale especially in the United States and in England. In time penicillin was obtained in sufficient quantity to enable its therapeutic possibilities to be widely explored and in a state of sufficient purity for its chemical composition to be determined.

Penicillin occurs in several isomeric forms, depending largely upon the type of culture used. It is an acid which forms salts with sodium, potassium, and calcium, these being official in the B.P. and U.S.P. They form light yellow or brownish powders, freely soluble in water. They are hygroscopic (especially the sodium salt) and must be kept in sealed containers. The activity of penicillin is expressed in Units per mg.

Benzylpenicillin, B.P., *Penicillin G*, U.S.P., a white crystalline powder of known constitutional formula $C_{16}H_{17}O_4N_2S$ Na (or K), is the official type for injection, though there is no restriction on the other types for topical application. The calcium salts of *Amorphous Penicillin*, B.P., are usually confined to external application and the crystalline sodium or potassium salts to injection.

The supreme value of penicillin rests in its action on pathogenic organisms, but it is still uncertain how exactly this action is produced. This may be merely bacteriostatic (i.e. inhibiting the multiplication of bacteria) or actively bactericidal (i.e. killing bacteria), depending upon the concentration of penicillin and the particular infection which is being treated. It is markedly selective in its action, susceptible organisms including most staphylococci and streptococci, pneumococcus, meningococcus, gonococcus, and the *Treponema pallidum* of syphilis. Many bacteria are resistant to it, including typhoid and tubercle bacilli. Generally, most Gram-negative organisms are resistant to it. When possible, it is advisable to ensure that an infecting organism is susceptible to it, otherwise time and material may be wasted in fruitless treatment.

Penicillin is widely used as a local antiseptic for wounds, mucous membranes, &c. To subserve these uses there are official B.P. preparations: *Ointment* and *Cream* for the skin; *Eye Ointment*; and *Lozenges* for the mouth and throat.

Its most important use is, however, as a systemic antiseptic, for which purpose it has acquired a pre-eminent and still growing reputation. Penicillin is rapidly but irregularly and inadequately absorbed when given by mouth because it is destroyed by the acid gastric juice and by penicillinase from coliform organisms. The advantages of an effective oral preparation are so obvious, particularly in treating children, that many attempts have been made to produce a stable, acid-resistant ester of penicillin. One such, phenoxymethyl penicillin, is relatively effective; it is produced by biosynthesis, that is to say, the culture medium in which the mould is growing is treated with a substrate hydroxyethyl-phenoxyacetamide, which is incorporated by the mould in the penicillin it produces. The dosage of this preparation is 125 mg. three or more times per day. Penicillin is, however, more rapidly (in about ten minutes) and completely absorbed when injected intramuscularly, and this is the usual channel of administration. For this purpose the *Injection of Penicillin*, B.P., a solution in sterile water, or *Buffered Crystalline Penicillin G*, U.S.P., can be used.

Distribution of absorbed penicillin in the body is widespread, but effective concentrations do not reach the cerebrospinal fluid. In meningitis it may be injected intrathecally. Penicillin is rapidly excreted in the urine and may have to be administered every 3 hours or so in order to maintain an effective concentration in the blood. Attempts have been made to delay the excretion of penicillin by giving agents such as caronamide which delay excretion, but these are not much favoured. The other approach to the problem is to administer an ester or other form of penicillin, a so-called depot preparation, from which slow absorption may take place. Formerly mixtures of penicillin in oil and wax were used; then it was discovered that the local anaesthetic procaine would combine with the antibiotic to produce a white precipitate. This substance is administered in suspension, subcutaneously or intramuscularly, as *Injection of Procaine Benzylpenicillin,* B.P., *Sterile Procaine Penicillin G Suspension*, U.S.P., and various other preparations of it are available. It liberates penicillin slowly, giving peak concentrations only after several hours and the excretion is accordingly delayed, so that it may be administered once or twice per day. Several of the biosynthetic esters, such as *Benzathine Penicillin G*, U.S.P., are also slowly absorbed and may be effective if given once daily.

Bacteria may become resistant to penicillin (p. 280); to avoid this occurrence, effective doses should be given early. It is impossible here to mention in detail all the diseases in the treatment of which it has proved so valuable. It is superior to all other remedies in staphylococcal infections, in gonorrhoea, and in syphilis. It has greatly diminished the death-rate in lobar pneumonia, where it is especially valuable if the pneumococci are resistant to sulphonamides (p. 272). It is very free from serious toxic effects, apart from those already mentioned.

Dosage must be adjusted to the needs of the patient, the nature, severity, and duration of the infection, but it is essential to realize that therapy with penicillin does not offer a substitute for surgical drainage of pus and debris nor does its use mean that other measures may be neglected. *Injection of Penicillin*, B.P., (Amorphous Penicillin or Benzylpenicillin), may be given in doses of 500,000–1,000,000 Units per day; 250,000 Units per ml. *Injection of Procaine Benzylpenicillin*, B.P., is given in similar dosage; 300,000 Units per ml. The U.S.P. prefers 200,000 U.S.P. Units, 4 times a day, for *Buffered Crystalline Penicillin G*, and 300,000 U.S.P. Units, once or twice a day for *Sterile Procaine Penicillin G Suspension*.

The success of pencillin prompted wider investigations which have shown that the property of elaborating bactericidal substances is by no means confined to *Penicillium notatum* but is widespread among fungi and even bacteria. Of the many substances which have been investigated, no one among this group has been discovered which rivals penicillin in range of therapeutic activity combined with low toxicity. The most promising so far are streptomycin, chloramphenicol, and the tetracyclines.

STREPTOMYCIN

Streptomycin is obtained from *Streptomyces griseus* grown in deep culture. It is a basic organic compound official as *Streptomycin Hydrochloride*, B.P., *Streptomycin Sulphate*, B.P., U.S.P., or *Streptomycin Calcium Chloride*, B.P., salts which are water-soluble. Taken by mouth it is not absorbed and must therefore be given parenterally (usually intramuscularly) or by topical application. Absorption is relatively slow, 2 hours passing before peak concentrations occur. It is distributed in the extracellular fluids only, and excreted within 12–14 hours. If renal function is impaired it may accumulate dangerously. It is partially excreted in tears, saliva, sweat, and milk, crosses the placental barrier, and may appear in the cerebrospinal fluid of patients with meningitis but not in that of normal persons. It is found in exudates but not readily in abscesses. *Dihydrostreptomycin*, B.P., (as sulphate or hydrochloride), *Dihydrostreptomycin Sulfate*, U.S.P., is a synthetic modification with similar properties. Streptomycin and dihydrostreptomycin are not usually toxic in therapeutic doses, but in susceptible persons and with high dosage the parent substance may damage the vestibular part of the eighth nerve, producing vertigo, and the synthetic product the auditory branch of that nerve producing deafness. It may sometimes be considered worthwhile, therefore, to use a mixture of the two, each in half the amount necessary for a full chemotherapeutic effect *Streptoduocin for Injection*, U.S.P. In addition, allergic responses occur, especially on contact with solutions of these antibiotics. Streptomycin is bacteriostatic and bactericidal and affects a wide range of organisms including most of those affected by penicillin but it is active against Gram-negative bacilli such as *Proteus, Pseudomonas, Aerobacter, Str. faecalis*, and particularly *Mycobacterium*. Unfortunately there is a strong tendency towards the development of resistant strains of these and other bacteria towards the two antibiotics, which limits their usefulness. Viomycin, a similar substance obtained from *Actinomyces*, has the same drawbacks but does not show cross-tolerance with streptomycin. Solutions of streptomycin for injection are somewhat unstable and are made up immediately before administration, as with penicillin. The potency of *Streptomycin Sulphate*, B.P., is 600 micrograms of pure base per mg. of material and the dose is usually 0·5–1 G. of base every 2–3 days for a period of as many weeks as necessary. In tuberculous meningitis daily injections are needed, at least for a time, and in addition 50–100 mg. may be given daily intrathecally.

TUBERCULOSTATIC DRUGS

The great facility with which the tubercle bacillus develops resistance to streptomycin led to disappointment in the results of treatment with this antibiotic alone. Meanwhile other types of synthetic antitubercular compound had been tried.

Sodium Aminosalicylate, B.P., *Aminosalicylic Acid*, U.S.P., (Para-aminosalicylic Acid, PAS), was investigated because it had been shown that benzoic and salicylic acids increased the metabolic activity of *Mycobacterium* and it was hoped that the salicylic analogue might interfere with some process essential to the organism. PAS is readily absorbed when given by mouth and is excreted in 12–24 hours in the urine. Its antibacterial activity is less than that of streptomycin when tested in cultures of tubercle bacilli but in the body the drugs are synergistic. Its main virtue is that when given in conjunction with the antibiotic it delays or prevents the appearance of drug resistance. Unfortunately it has to be given in massive doses—20 G. per day —which often cause nausea, vomiting, diarrhoea, or mental depression.

Isoniazid, B.P., U.S.P., is a synthetic drug of simple structure.

Isoniazid.

It is readily absorbed, reaches peak levels after oral administration in 1–2 hours, and is acetylated and excreted in the urine fairly rapidly. The drug is widely diffused and tends to concentrate in the skin and in the internal organs, including the lungs. It penetrates caseous material and reaches tuberculous foci and abscesses. *In vitro* this substance is much more active against *Myco. tuberculosis* than is streptomycin. It is highly specific, being ineffective against most other organisms. In patients it exerts a rather delayed bacteriostatic action. The mode of action is not precisely understood but in doses of 0·1–0·3 G. daily, in conjunction either with streptomycin or PAS, it is a highly effective treatment in all forms of tuberculosis. Toxicity is relatively slight—some episodes of allergy, gastrointestinal upset, rarely depression of the bone marrow.

These drugs, given usually as combinations of the antibiotic with one or both synthetic compounds, less frequently as PAS —isoniazid combinations without antibiotic, have reduced the disability and mortality from tuberculosis.

CHLORAMPHENICOL

Chloramphenicol is a halogenated nitrobenzene compound originally derived from culture of *Streptomyces venezuelae*, but now synthesized—the first antibiotic to be so produced on a commercial scale. It is relatively insoluble and has to be given by mouth, though a suspension is available for intramuscular injection. It is absorbed quite readily after oral administration, reaching high blood levels in 2 hours. It is distributed widely, penetrating into the cells, crossing the placenta, and appearing in exudates, abscesses, cerebrospinal fluid, &c. It is excreted in a few hours by the kidney in inactive form. It may cause nausea and vomiting, occasional allergy, especially from topical application, and there is a risk of suppression of bone marrow activity with consequent blood dyscrasia, which has proved fatal on occasion. This antibiotic is active against many Gram-negative bacteria and in addition inhibits the rickettsiae and a few viruses. It is probably the drug of choice in treating typhus fever, scrub typhus, Rocky Mountain spotted fever, Q. fever, &c., and typhoid fever. It is less effective in paratyphoid fevers but is of great value in psittacosis and lymphogranuloma. It is given in 0·25 G. capsules, 1·5–4 G. per day, as needed, and should not be continued any longer than is strictly necessary. The official preparations are *Chloramphenicol*, B.P., U.S.P., the *Capsules*, B.P., U.S.P., and the *Ophthalmic Ointment*, U.S.P.

THE TETRACYCLINES

The Tetracyclines are a group of antibiotics produced by related species of *Streptomyces*. They are *Tetracycline*, U.S.P., *Aureomycin Hydrochloride*, B.P., (*Chlortetracycline*, U.S.P.), and *Oxytetracycline*, B.P., U.S.P., (Terramycin). Tetracycline is the most soluble and stable, chlortetracycline the least stable and brightest yellow in colour. They have a bitter taste like chloramphenicol and are given by mouth in tablets or capsules of 0·25 G. The potency is usually 900 Units of activity per mg. Absorption after oral administration is good, peak blood levels being reached in 2–4 hours. Chlortetracycline is largely bound to tissue protein. Distribution is widespread and includes penetration into cells and cerebrospinal fluid. Tetracycline is perhaps the most effective in passing the blood-brain barrier. Excretion is partly in urine and partly into the intestine. The tetracyclines have a very wide antibacterial spectrum which includes Gram-positive and Gram-negative bacteria, rickettsiae, some viruses, spirochaetes, *Myco. tuberculosis* to a variable degree, and to some extent *Entamoeba histolytica*, the causative organism of amoebic dysentery. These drugs produce bacteriostatic and bactericidal effects by interfering with the synthesis of protein in rapidly growing organisms. They are given orally as *Capsules* or *Tablets* in doses of 1–2 G. daily of *Aureomycin Hydrochloride*, B.P.; 1–4 G. daily of *Oxytetracycline Dihydrate*, B.P., or 1 Gm. daily of any U.S.P. tetracycline. Chlortetracycline and oxytetracycline as hydrochlorides may be injected. They produce remarkably little toxicity, perhaps some gastrointestinal upset. They are of value in treating penicillin-resistant infections, for brucellosis, typhus fevers, obscure pneumonias and broncho-pneumonias, and many other conditions. *Ophthalmic Ointments*, U.S.P., are available.

OTHER ANTIBIOTICS

Bacitracin, U.S.P., is a polypeptide material extracted from cultures of a *Bacillus subtilis* species. This substance is not absorbed if taken by mouth but may be given by all parenteral routes or applied topically. It is active against a wide range of Gram-positive and Gram-negative organisms, spirochaetes, and clostridia of gas-gangrene. It is of value in the treatment of penicillin-resistant infections and is often applied topically for the treatment of furunculosis, &c. Injected intramuscularly it is readily absorbed and excreted in 6–8 hours. It has some toxic effect on the kidney, diuresis, with albumin and casts often occurring, but though this situation needs care it is not a clear indication for withdrawal of the drug, as the evidence of renal damage soon disappears with continuing dosage. Some 10,000 Units may be given 8-hourly to an adult by injection. Bacitracin is painful on injection and may be mixed with a solution of procaine but this practice is to be avoided when the antibiotic is used by local instillation in the treatment of infections of the central nervous system and adjacent structures. The *Ointment*, U.S.P., contains 500 U./G.

Erythromycin, U.S.P., is a rather insoluble, bitter-tasting antibiotic obtained from *Streptomyces erythreus*. The constitution is not yet determined. It is very similar in its antibacterial activity to penicillin and is often reserved for the treatment of penicillin-resistant staphylococcal and other infections. When applied topically it may give rise to sensitization phenomena; oral administration has caused gastro-intestinal upsets but on the whole it is not toxic nor does it cause profound changes in the intestinal flora. It is administered in 200 mg. *Tablets*, U.S.P., in a dosage of 200–600 mg. 6-hourly.

Neomycin Sulfate, U.S.P., is the soluble salt of a base with antibiotic properties obtained from *Streptomyces fradiae*. It differs from other antibiotics in being extremely stable, resisting heat and alkalinization. The antibacterial spectrum is wider than that of penicillin and streptomycin and it may be effective against penicillin-resistant staphylococci and Gram-negative infections such as *Haemophilus*, &c. It may be injected intramuscularly, not more than 1 Gm. per day. Overdosage may produce damage to the kidney or the eighth nerve. It may be applied topically for the cure of indolent ulcers and resistant superficial infections. It is given by mouth in doses of 4–10 Gm. per day for a few days in order partially to sterilize the lower bowel before surgery of these parts but such a procedure may give rise to diarrhoea or be the cause of an efflorescence of yeasts and resistant organisms. It is very poorly absorbed from the gastro-intestinal tract. The *Tablet* and *Ointment* are official in U.S.P.

Polymyxin B Sulfate, U.S.P., is one of a mixture of substances produced by *Bacillus polymyxa* (*aerosporus*). It is a polypeptide base, stable in solution, and actively bactericidal against Gram-negative bacteria such as *Bact. coli*, *Pseudomonas*, &c. *Proteus* is often resistant. This antibiotic is toxic to the kidney and to the nervous system in overdosage but may be administered intrathecally in case of necessity. Given by mouth it is of value in the treatment of *Shigella* dysentery, and topically may be applied to the skin or the eye. The potency is 6,000 U./mg. and the daily dose by injection should not exceed 500 mg. given in divided doses of 750,000 U.S.P. Units four times a day. Procaine may be mixed with it if it is not being used in or near the central nervous system. It is not recoverable from the urine, apparently being bound to tissue protein.

INFECTIONS OF THE URINARY PASSAGES

Infections of the urethra or of the bladder may be treated locally by antiseptic injections, but infections of the urinary passages generally, including the kidney (pyelitis), can also be treated by drugs given by mouth, which are absorbed and excreted by the kidney.

Methenamine, U.S.P., (Hexamine), $(CH_2)_6N_4$, is a condensation product of ammonia and formaldehyde. By itself hexamine is not antiseptic, and produces no marked physiological actions. When given by mouth, it is excreted in the urine, and, if this is acid, is decomposed with the liberation of formaldehyde, which is a powerful antiseptic. It has no such action if the urine is alkaline. It is given in doses of 1 Gm. four times a day. If the urine is not sufficiently acid, acid sodium phosphate or ammonium chloride has to be given as well. It is generally inferior to sulphonamides and mandelates.

Among other substances which exert an antiseptic action on the urine when given by the mouth may be mentioned mandelic acid $(C_6H_5 \cdot CHOH \cdot COOH)$ and hexylresorcinol (p. 307).

Mandelic acid is bactericidal only in acid urine. As it is irritating to the stomach the less irritating *Calcium Mandelate*, U.S.P., (3 Gm. four times a day), is preferred to the free acid. Ammonium chloride is also given to make the urine acid. The salt ammonium mandelate may also be used.

Methenamine Mandelate, U.S.P., is given in doses of 1 Gm. up to four times a day and combines to some extent the actions of hexamine and mandelic acid.

Recently the sulphonamides have been extensively used as urinary antiseptics. For most infections *Sulfisoxazole*, U.S.P.,

(Sulphafurazole), appears to be suitable, though any of the systemic sulphonamides are effective.

Several of the antibiotics are of great value—streptomycin for tuberculous and Gram-negative infections such as *E. coli*, and the tetracyclines for Gram-positive infections. It must always be remembered that the primary necessity is a clear passage for the urine; any form of stasis must be dealt with if permanent success is to be achieved.

XXV

DRUGS USED IN PROTOZOAL INFECTIONS

TRYPANOSOMIASIS

MANY important diseases, occurring in man and in domesticated and wild animals, are due to infection by organisms of the trypanosome type, including spirochaetes. Infection is usually produced by contact or by the bite of an insect. Trypanosome infections lend themselves readily to chemotherapeutic investigation because certain species of trypanosomes are readily communicable (e.g. by injection of blood from an infected animal) to small animals. The organisms are readily detected in the blood, and their number gives an indication of the severity of the infection. A suitable remedy causes reduction or disappearance of the organisms in the blood and prolongs the life of the animal. The therapeutic value of a substance can, therefore, be rapidly determined.

A remedy which is successful for a disease due to one particular trypanosome will probably be more or less efficacious against other trypanosomes or against spirochaetes, because these organisms are closely allied. The resistance of different species of trypanosomes to a particular therapeutic agent may, however, vary considerably, and the toxicity of the latter for different animals may also vary. Consequently the final estimate of the value of a remedy (and this applies to all remedies and all infections) must be made with regard to disease due to a specific organism and occurring in the particular species of animal to be cured.

Generally speaking (and this is true of most, if not all, infections) the prospect of cure is greater the earlier in the disease the remedy is given, mainly because in the early stages of an infection the organisms have had less time to multiply or to invade less accessible regions. When, for example, trypanosomes or spirochaetes have invaded the central nervous system, remedies which would have been efficacious in earlier stages of the disease may fail to act.

Drugs which are used in the treatment of syphilis and trypanosomiasis have already been considered. They include mercury (p. 60), bismuth (p. 68), arsenic (p. 71), antimony (p. 69), certain dyes, and penicillin (p. 281).

Two types of chemical compounds were found by Ehrlich to give promising results in the treatment of experimental trypanosomiasis in lower animals, namely, organic arsenical compounds and certain dyes. Researches on the former group have led to the introduction of arsphenamine, tryparsamide, &c. Of substances belonging to the class of trypanocidal dyes one, *Suramin*, B.P., has been used in the prophylaxis and treatment of sleeping sickness. Its precise method of action is not known. It is effective especially in the early stages of the disease before the organisms have invaded the central nervous system. It has no action on trypanosomes *in vitro*, but a single injection can produce a prolonged immunity to infection by them. It may produce toxic effects, especially on the kidney. It is especially useful in the treatment of trypanosomiasis when the parasites are resistant to tryparsamide. Dose, by intravenous injection, 1–2 G.

The trypanocidal action of another group of compounds, more recently introduced, was discovered in the following way. Synthalin and its parent substance, guanidine, have the property of lowering blood sugar. Synthalin was found to have a therapeutic effect in mice infected with trypanosomes, and it was supposed at first that this effect might be due to the reduction in blood sugar, for trypanosomes are very sensitive to a reduction in the sugar content of the medium in which they live. Later it was found that synthalin had a direct action on trypanosomes. This finding stimulated investigation of compounds related to synthalin. Of these, three especially have been tried clinically: *Stilbamidine*, *Pentamidine*, and *Propamidine*. They have been found useful in early stages of trypanosomiasis and especially in leishmaniasis. They are usually given intramuscularly or intravenously as isothianates.

Of diseases due to amoeboid organisms two require specific mention, not only because of the importance of the diseases themselves, but from the successful curative results that have been achieved in them by the use of chemical remedies.

MALARIA

Malaria is one of the most important of all diseases, because millions of people suffer from it in various parts of the world and it is responsible for a high rate of ill health and mortality. The disease is due to a protozoal parasite which gains entrance into the human body by the bite of an infected mosquito. The parasites as injected by the mosquito are thin, nucleated rods, called 'sporozoites'. These sporozoites enter the liver and other reticulo-endothelial cells and there undergo development during an incubation period of a few days to a few weeks, preliminary to invading the erythrocytes—the exo-erythrocytic stage of the life-cycle. They then enter the red blood corpuscles and therein undergo a series of changes, finally undergoing sporulation into merozoites, the number of which (6–20) varies with the species of malarial parasite. The merozoites rupture the corpuscle and escape into the plasma, and later enter the corpuscles again and continue this asexual cycle of changes, which can persist indefinitely until the disease is cured. In time some develop into sexual forms, gametocytes. If a mosquito ingests blood containing gametocytes, these undergo a sexual cycle in the mosquito, leading ultimately to the formation of sporozoites which, if injected into a human host by the bite of a mosquito, start the asexual cycle above described.

It is the asexual cycle of the parasite that causes the symptoms of the disease in man. At each time of the liberation of merozoites from the ruptured corpuscles, a steep rise of temperature occurs, with other symptoms characteristic of malarial fever. These symptoms occur only when there are a sufficient number of parasites in the blood and, after inoculation, there is a symptomless incubation period (usually about a fortnight) until this number is reached.

The exo-erythrocytic forms of the parasite which are developed in the liver during this incubation period may remain in the liver independently of the blood cycle and later invade the erythrocytes causing relapses of acute malaria. They are probably less easily reached by a drug and also more resistant to its action than are the erythrocytic forms. Hence a drug may destroy the latter but not the former, and therefore be capable of suppressing acute attacks without preventing subsequent relapses, especially if the drug is discontinued. Relapses occur especially with *Plasmodium vivax*, the commonest type of malaria.

There are three main types of malaria in man, each due to a different parasite: benign tertian malaria (*Plasmodium vivax*), malignant tertian malaria (*P. falciparum*), and quartan malaria (*P. malariae*). According to the type of malarial parasite, the asexual cycle occupies either two or three days, and, as the fever coincides with the liberation of merozoites, there is an attack of fever every two or three days, in tertian and quartan malaria respectively. The fever subsides after a few hours, the temperature being normal between attacks.

With this brief account of the disease, there are certain problems connected with malarial fevers that can be readily understood. The *treatment* of attacks of malaria in man consists in destroying the parasites in the tissues, which will give a complete cure, or in reducing their number to below that which causes symptoms. This can be done with quinine and other drugs to be mentioned. The *prophylaxis* of malaria could be achieved by preventing persons being bitten by mosquitoes (e.g. by the use of mosquito-proof gauzes or insect repellents) or by administering a drug which would prevent the development of the parasite when it was injected by mosquito bite. The *eradication* of malaria in a district would occur if mosquitoes or their larvae could be destroyed, or if there were no persons with malarial gametocytes in their peripheral blood, because, unless these are ingested by the mosquito, the life-cycle of the parasite cannot be continued. All these methods of combating the disease are being tried with greater or less success.

Man is not the only animal to harbour parasites of the malarial type. Similar organisms, more or less pathogenic, are found in many mammals and birds. Birds, e.g. canaries, can be inoculated with a type of malaria to which they are susceptible; and in recent years a technique has been developed whereby the potential value of new chemical compounds can be estimated by their efficacy in curing malaria in birds.

A remedy efficacious in bird malaria may not be equally effective in human malaria, or vice versa; but nevertheless, with the facility of experimentation provided by bird malaria, chemotherapeutic investigation has led to the discovery of new remedies for human malaria, e.g. mepacrine and proguanil.

QUININE

Quinine is found in the bark of various species of cinchona, which are natives of South America but are now cultivated also in the East. Cinchona bark was introduced into European medicine in the middle of the seventeenth century, and its name was derived from the Countess of Cinchon who was successfully treated by it in the earliest years of its use. Quinine was isolated from the bark in 1820, since when the use of the pure alkaloid has gradually replaced that of preparations of the crude bark. Cinchona bark contains a large number of alkaloids, about one-half of the total amount being quinine. Generally, the other alkaloids resemble quinine in constitution and action, but none of them equal it in importance. Quinine has a complicated structural formula which includes a quinoline and a quinuclidine group.

A distinguishing feature of the action of quinine is the relatively low concentrations of it that diminish the activity and vitality of certain protozoal organisms. It is owing to this property that it acts so successfully in malaria. Quinine destroys the parasite and therefore the fever disappears. Some types of malaria are more favourably influenced by quinine than others. If all the parasites are killed, the malaria is cured; but often, though the parasites disappear from the peripheral blood, they may persist elsewhere in the body in more resistant forms and after a variable period there may be a relapse of malaria, especially if the administration of quinine be discontinued. A common dosage in malaria is 1·8 G. (30 gr.) of quinine a day for a few days, afterwards reduced to 0·6 G. (10 gr.), a day. It may also be taken nightly, 0·3 G. (5 gr.) as a suppressive to ward off clinical symptoms without actually curing the disease. Though quinine has been largely superseded by newer remedies, some still regard quinine, administered parenterally, as the drug of choice in cerebral malaria.

Quinine is much less effective as an antipyretic in fevers other than malaria, and in these its action has not been satisfactorily explained. Quinine not only interferes with the vitality of living organisms but also hinders the action of unorganized ferments, e.g. the oxidizing ferments of the blood. Possibly as the result of this action it seems to diminish the metabolism of cells generally. It acts as an antipyretic also by a central action. In most fevers, however, it is not so efficient an antipyretic as the members of the phenacetin group.

Of the other pharmacological actions of quinine, that on voluntary muscle has been mentioned (p. 150). Quinine depresses the activity of ciliated epithelium and also, like quinidine, cardiac irritability. Low concentrations, such as occur in the blood after medicinal doses, may cause increased contraction of involuntary muscle, especially of the spleen or uterus. It has been used to promote uterine contractions in labour, but it is not comparable in power to pituitary or ergot.

Large doses, or continued maximal therapeutic doses, produce disturbances of the senses of hearing and sight; ringing in the ears, deafness, vertigo, and contraction of the field of vision (*cinchonism*). Usually these effects are transient and disappear when the quinine is discontinued. Fatal cases of poisoning are very rare when quinine is given by mouth. Intravenously, it must be given with care (well diluted and slowly injected), otherwise it may cause respiratory and cardiac failure.

There is very marked idiosyncrasy to quinine, for some few

people suffer from disorders of hearing and sight as the result of much smaller doses than produce these symptoms in the great majority of people. In others, skin rashes are produced.

An important contra-indication to the use of quinine is in blackwater fever, a serious complication of malaria (especially of chronic *P. falciparum* infections) in which rapid haemolysis of the red cells in the blood leads to haemoglobinuria ('blackwater'). The use of quinine especially in inadequate doses is a predisposing or exciting factor. Fortunately newer remedies like mepacrine do not have this effect, and blackwater fever has almost disappeared since they have replaced quinine in the treatment of this type of infection.

Cinchona contains a large number of alkaloids, of which quinine, quinidine, cinchonine, and cinchonidine are best known. These resemble one another in constitution and actions and all have some action in malaria, but none has proved superior to quinine. Several salts of quinine are in use. *Quinine Sulphate*, B.P., U.S.P., forms light feathery crystals, with intensely bitter taste, soluble 1 in 800 in water. It can be dissolved by addition of an acid, and dilute sulphuric acid is often used for this purpose in mixtures. *Quinine Bisulphate*, B.P., soluble 1 in 10, *Quinine Hydrochloride*, B.P., U.S.P., (1 in 32), or especially *Quinine Dihydrochloride*, B.P., (1 in 1) can be used when a more soluble salt is advisable.

S UBSTITUTES FOR QUININE

The need for substitutes for quinine became imperative when in 1942 the Japanese gained control of Java, which up to then was supplying 90 per cent. of the world's quinine requirements. Campaigning in a highly malarial district was impossible without a malaria-suppressant, owing to the high incapacity and mortality rates among the soldiers. Fortunately new antimalarials were discovered, even more effective than quinine. They act on different forms of the malarial parasite and can be so classified. It is important to distinguish them, as their differences determine their appropriate uses.

1. ACTING ON ERYTHROCYTIC FORMS. These resemble

quinine in having no effective action either on the exo-erythro-cytic forms of the parasite or on the gametocytes. They act on the erythrocytic forms which are responsible for the attacks of malarial fever. They are used in two ways: (*a*) To abort existing attacks of malarial fever, that is for the 'clinical cure' of the symptoms (not necessarily or usually a radical cure of the disease). Such a drug may be called a *therapeutic suppressant*. (*b*) To prevent febrile attacks ever occurring in spite of possible exposure to infection. This it does by preventing erythrocytic forms developing in sufficient numbers to provoke fever. Used in this way the drug can be called a *suppressive prophylactic*.

It is a fairly general rule with chemotherapeutic remedies that they act the more effectively the smaller the number of patho-genic organisms they have to contend with. Consequently smaller doses are required for prophylaxis than for aborting acute attacks but these smaller doses have to be given con-tinuously to prevent overt febrile symptoms developing in per-sons who have been bitten by an infected mosquito.

Mepacrine Hydrochloride, B.P., called **Quinacrine Hydro-chloride**, U.S.P., is a bright yellow powder with a bitter taste. It is at least as effective as quinine in suppressing attacks of malarial fever and, by taking small daily doses, it is possible to live in a highly malarious district without getting overt attacks of malaria. It may produce yellowness of the skin which disappears within a few days or weeks after the drug is discontinued. Occasional toxic symptoms include headache, abdominal pain, or, rarely, mental symptoms. Dose, prophy-lactic, 0·1 G. daily; therapeutic 0·2–0·5 G. daily in divided doses. It is also an effective agent for expelling tapeworms (p. 306).

Chloroquine Phosphate, B.P., U.S.P., is colourless, bitter, and soluble, and does not discolour the skin like mepacrine. It resembles quinine and mepacrine in that its action is limited to the erythrocytic forms of the parasite and like them it can cure an acute attack of *P. falciparum* fever and suppress that due to *P. vivax*, for which a total dose of 2·5 G. in 3 days is usually sufficient. It is an excellent suppressive prophylactic, having the advantage that, owing to its slow excretion, it need be given only once a week, in a dose of 0·5 G. Chloroquine is also used in amoebic dysentery (p. 304).

Amodiaquine (Camoquin) is very similar to chloroquine both as a suppressant and as a prophylactic.

2. ACTING ON EXO-ERYTHROCYTIC AND ERYTHROCYTIC FORMS.

The second group of antimalarials has an action on the erythrocytic forms of parasite but has in addition a lethal effect on exo-erythrocytic forms. Owing to the former action they can suppress attacks of malarial fever like quinine and mepacrine; owing to the latter action they can also destroy parasites latent in the liver which cause relapses of malaria; for which reason they are called *causal prophylactics*.

Proguanil Hydrochloride, B.P., (Paludrine), is colourless, bitter, and sparingly soluble. It is an effective suppressant, especially against *P. falciparum* infections. It is slower in action than chloroquine which is preferable for treatment of acute attacks. Proguanil has been extensively and successfully used as a causal prophylactic. It is very free from toxic effects. Some strains of malaria acquire a resistance to it, which may limit its usefulness. The dosage ranges from 0·1 G. to 0·4 G. daily.

Pyrimethamine is chemically related to proguanil and has very similar actions but is more active and less likely to give rise to resistant strains. The dosage is very small: 5 mg. weekly as a suppressive prophylactic, 5 mg. daily as a causal prophylactic, and 100 mg. for treatment of an acute attack.

3. ACTING ON GAMETOCYTES AND EXO-ERYTHROCYTIC FORMS.

The third group of antimalarials have little or no action on the erythrocytic forms of malarial parasite and have therefore no effect in curing acute attacks; on the other hand they destroy some of the exo-erythrocytic forms and also the gametocytes.

Pamaquin, B.P., 10–20 mg., is chiefly used in combination with a schizonticidal drug like chloroquine to prevent relapses and effect a radical cure of *P. vivax* malaria. It destroys the gametocytes or renders them incapable of reproduction. Hence it could be used to interrupt the life-cycle of the parasite by stopping the infection of the mosquito and so to prevent the spread of malaria. Pamaquin is, however, a rather toxic as well as expensive substance and there are obvious difficulties in administering it in sufficient doses to all the people in a district who may be infected with malaria. Among the toxic symptoms which may occur with pamaquin are epigastric pain, cyanosis, methaemoglobinaemia, cardiac arrhythmia, and liver necrosis.

Primaquine Phosphate, U.S.P., is related structurally to pamaquin and has similar actions and uses. It is less toxic than pamaquin which it has now largely replaced.

AMOEBIC DYSENTERY

This disease, like malaria, is due to an amoeboid organism, which is, however, probably not very closely related to the malarial organism. In any case quinine has but little effect on amoebic dysentery, and conversely ipecacuanha, the actions of which may here be considered, has little or no beneficial action in malaria.

The term 'dysentery' is merely a symptomatic name to designate a disorder of the intestines characterized by the frequent passage of blood and mucus from the bowel, usually accompanied by pain and tenesmus, often with severe inflammation and ulceration of the colon. Such symptoms can be produced by different types of infection. There are two main types of dysentery, bacillary and amoebic, which require different treatments. Mention has already been made of the treatment of bacillary dysentery (p. 277).

IPECACUANHA

Ipecacuanha is the dried root of *Cephaëlis ipecacuanha*, a small shrub which grows in Brazil. It began to be imported into Europe in the seventeenth century as a remedy for dysentery. For this it has been used more or less continuously since, at first with varying success, but with more certain results in recent years since it has been realized that it is only in one particular form of dysentery—that due to amoebic infection—that it has a curative action. In the course of time it has acquired other therapeutic uses.

The active principles of ipecacuanha root are alkaloids, of which the most important is emetine. Emetine has a peculiar irritant action which it can display even on the skin, but more conspicuously on mucous membranes. The first group of actions to be described are the result of this irritant action. Thus when taken by mouth in doses of about 1 G. (15 gr.), of the powdered root, ipecacuanha produces vomiting reflexly through irritation of the mucous membranes of the stomach. Vomiting is slow in onset and accompanied by much nausea, and is apt to be repeated. Where speedy emesis is desirable, e.g. in cases of poisoning, ipecacuanha is therefore unsuitable.

It is more often used for effects which accompany gastric irritation, namely increased bronchial and sweat secretion. The degree of irritation necessary to produce increased bronchial secretion is something short of that necessary to evoke vomiting. Hence doses of ipecacuanha, e.g. about 1 gr., too small to produce vomiting, can cause increased secretion from the bronchial mucous membrane. This effect can be produced similarly by other gastric irritants, e.g. tartar emetic, ammonium carbonate, squill, &c. Many such substances can therefore be used as expectorants, and their method of action has been described in greater detail on p. 199. Preparations of ipecacuanha commonly used for this purpose are *Tincture of Ipecacuanha*, B.P., in doses of 0·6–2 ml. (10–30 min.), or *Ipecac Syrup*, U.S.P., in doses of 8 ml. To produce vomiting with these preparations about ten times as much must be given.

A second accompaniment of gastric irritation is increased sweating. This is produced reflexly in much the same way as increased bronchial secretion, and indeed a cold sweat is a well-known concomitant of nausea from any cause.

A famous powder used for this purpose is *Powder of Ipecacuanha and Opium* or Dover's Powder. The originator of this powder, Thomas Dover, was a romantic figure. If he had not turned buccaneer for a few years the story of Robinson Crusoe would never have been written, for it was Captain Thomas Dover on the privateer *Duke* who rescued Alexander Selkirk in 1709 after he had lived alone on an island for over four years, and whose story Defoe later wrote. Returning with a ship full of treasure in 1710, Dover at the age of forty began the practice of medicine with no qualifications other than that he had been at one time a servant of Sydenham. Perhaps his chief legacy to medicine was the powder which still bears his name. This powder, as now compounded, contains 10 per cent. each of ipecacuanha and opium, lactose making up the bulk of the powder. It is an efficient diaphoretic, ipecacuanha increasing the secretion of sweat—an effect which is enhanced by the dilatation of the skin vessels produced by opium. The dose is 0·3–0·6 G. (5–10 gr.). Dover's Powder has to some extent been supplanted by newer diaphoretics and antipyretics such as aspirin.

The most important therapeutic use of ipecacuanha is in a type of dysentery, especially prevalent in tropical countries, due to infection with a particular amoeba, *Entamoeba histolytica*. This amoeba infects the intestine, but may migrate from the intestinal canal and produce abscesses in the liver. The earliest use of ipecacuanha was in this disease, and it used to be given by mouth. In recent years it has been found that a more rapid and complete cure can be effected by administering the active principle emetine.

Emetine Hydrochloride, B.P., U.S.P., is given hypodermically or intramuscularly in a daily dose of 30–60 mg. ($\frac{1}{2}$–1 gr.), for several days. In many cases the amoebae disappear from the stools and liver, and the symptoms of the disease disappear. Emetine acts by killing the amoeba. This is the best treatment for the acute attack, and usually soon brings the diarrhoea under control, but it only effects a permanent cure in a minority of cases and should never be the only drug used in treating the disease. Emetine in the form of *Emetine and Bismuth Iodide*, B.P., (an insoluble salt which is not decomposed to liberate emetine until it reaches the intestine) is given by mouth in daily doses of 60–200 mg. (1–3 gr.) for about ten days, after the injections of emetine have ceased. This is also often effective in the more chronic forms of dysentery which are not cured by hypodermic injections of emetine. Toxic effects, e.g. neuritis and dilatation of the heart, may occur from repeated high dosage of emetine.

In cases where emetine treatment fails to eradicate the disease, several other remedies can be used to supplement its action. Organic arsenical compounds, *Acetarsol*, B.P., and *Carbarsone*, B.P., U.S.P., can be given by mouth in conjunction with emetine. Some quinoline derivatives, e.g. *Chiniofon Sodium*, B.P., *Chiniofon*, U.S.P., (0·1–0·5 G. orally, 1–5 G. by rectal injection) and *Di-iodohydroxyquinoline*, B.P., *Diiodohydroxyquin*, U.S.P., are of value. A combination of emetine with chloroquine (p. 299) has proved very successful in amoebic hepatitis and liver abscess. Chloroquine can be injected into the abscess cavity after drainage.

XXVI

DRUGS USED AS ANTHELMINTICS AND INSECTICIDES

ANTHELMINTICS

A VARIETY of diseases, some of great practical importance, especially in tropical and subtropical countries, are due to infection by worms. Here we have to deal with parasites far more highly organized, though not always more potent for ill, than the lowly protozoa or spirochaetes. It will not be surprising that, for diseases due to two groups of parasites phylogenetically so remote from one another, different remedies are usually necessary.

In some cases worms inhabit the tissues of the host. This is the case, for example, with bilharzia and filaria. These will be discussed later. In other cases the adult worm lives in the alimentary canal of the host, and drugs used to expel intestinal worms may be taken here. A drug used against worm infection is called an anthelmintic. If the worms are killed, it may be also called a vermicide. An anthelmintic may cause expulsion of live worms from the intestine, in which case the term vermifuge is preferable.

Different kinds of worms may be found in the intestine and, as they belong to different species, the same anthelmintic is not equally toxic to all. Frequently more than one anthelmintic is in use for any particular worm, so that it is convenient to group the anthelmintics according to the variety of worm for which each is chiefly used. It must be remembered, however, that the vermifuges so grouped together may have little in common, chemically or pharmacologically, beyond this anthelmintic action.

The attempt to get rid of intestinal worms will usually be successful only if attention be paid to details of treatment. It is generally advisable, before giving an anthelmintic, to have the stomach and intestine fairly empty of contents, so as to ensure access of the anthelmintic to the worm, without the drug being too diluted. This can be attained by keeping the patient on a light fluid diet on the previous day and by giving a purge. After the anthelmintic has had time to produce its effect it is usual to follow it with a second purgative, in order to remove any unabsorbed part of the drug, as well as to effect evacuation of dead or paralysed worms.

TAPEWORMS

Male Fern, B.P., *Aspidium*, U.S.P., the rhizome of a species of fern widely distributed over temperate regions, has been used for centuries as a vermifuge for tapeworm and is still a favourite drug for this purpose. The active principles are insoluble in water, and the preparation of male fern chiefly used is an ether extract, *Extract of Male Fern*, B.P., or *Aspidium Oleoresin*, U.S.P., a viscid oily-looking preparation which is administered in *Capsules* or suspended in mucilage in doses of 3–6 ml. (45–90 min.). The active principles are highly toxic if absorbed, but owing to their insolubility the extract does not usually cause toxic symptoms. In cases of unusual absorption or over-dosage the extract may produce gastro-intestinal irritation, with vomiting, diarrhoea, and abdominal pain, or in more severe cases convulsions or coma. Optic neuritis, leading to temporary or, rarely, permanent blindness, has occurred.

Mepacrine Hydrochloride, B.P., *Quinacrine Hydrochloride*, U.S.P., better known as a remedy for malaria (p. 299), is very effective in expelling tapeworms and may prove the best drug for the purpose. It is given in a single large dose of 15 mg./kg. (1 G. for an average adult) before breakfast with a saline purgative.

ROUNDWORMS

For infection by the common roundworm (*Ascaris lumbricoides*) the usual remedy is *Santonin*, B.P., a crystalline naphthalene derivative, obtained from the flower-heads of *Artemisia cina*. Santonin forms colourless crystals, which turn yellow on exposure to sunlight. It is almost insoluble in water, but soluble in alkalis. The roundworms are not killed by santonin but are expelled alive. Santonin is given in doses of 60–200 mg. (1–3 gr.). It is not now in the U.S.P.

Most of the santonin passes through the alimentary canal unabsorbed, the small amount excreted in the urine giving it a yellowish colour, or pinkish if alkaline. When absorbed in considerable quantities, santonin produces disorders of colour vision, yellow vision (xanthopsia) sometimes preceded by violet vision, due to an interference with violet perception in the retina. Santonin may also produce nausea and vomiting and, if absorbed in large quantities, epileptiform convulsions due to cerebral stimulation.

Hexylresorcinol, U.S.P., is another effective remedy against roundworms, dose 1 Gm.; for a child 100 mg. per year of age.

THREADWORMS

These are small worms which usually inhabit the rectum and can often be dislodged by rectal injections, e.g. of *Infusion of Quassia*, B.P., or of soap and water. If these measures fail to effect complete removal, other anthelmintics may be given by mouth. Among these are *Crystal Violet*, B.P., 10–30 mg. ($\frac{1}{6}$–$\frac{1}{2}$ gr.), *Methylrosaniline Chloride*, U.S.P., 60 mg. 3 times a day (p. 251), and *Diphenan*, B.P., 0·5–1 G. (8–15 gr.). A more recent introduction, piperazine adipate, produces a more rapid and complete cure of threadworm infestation and is free from serious side-effects and from staining properties. It is also effective against roundworms and pinworms.

HOOKWORMS

These are small nematodes, not over half an inch long, which live in the jejunum. There are at least two varieties, *Ankylostoma duodenale* or Old World hookworm, and *Necator americanus* or New World hookworm. In certain regions hookworm infection is very prevalent and responsible for much ill health, especially a form of progressive anaemia, so that the treatment of such infection is of great practical importance. The chief remedies are chenopodium oil, carbon tetrachloride, and tetrachloroethylene.

Chenopodium Oil, B.P., is a crude volatile oil obtained from *Chenopodium anthelminticum*, a weed growing widely in the United States and which was used as a domestic remedy for infection by worms. It is especially effective against *Ankylostoma*, dose 0·2–1 ml. (3–15 min.). Toxic symptoms which may occur are giddiness and vomiting and, in severe cases, coma.

Carbon Tetrachloride, B.P., tetrachloromethane, CCl_4, which resembles chloroform in some ways in its action, has been used since 1921 as a remedy for hookworm. It is a colourless volatile liquid with a characteristic odour and burning taste, almost insoluble in water. It is unsafe in alcoholics or in persons with calcium deficiency. Like thymol, it is more effective against *Necator americanus* than against *Ankylostoma duodenale*. It is given as a single dose of 2–4 ml. (30–60 min.). Nausea, vomiting, giddiness, and drowsiness may follow its use. It may produce extensive fatty degeneration of the liver.

Oil of chenopodium and carbon tetrachloride, while effective remedies, are both liable to produce toxic symptoms, and have now been discarded by the U.S.P. (though still official in the B.P.) in favour of a compound, chemically nearly related to carbon tetrachloride—tetrachloroethylene.

Tetrachloroethylene, B.P., U.S.P., $Cl_2C \cdot CCl_2$, resembles carbon tetrachloride in its properties, but, though possibly no more powerfully anthelmintic than carbon tetrachloride, it is less readily absorbed and less toxic. Many authorities consider that the most satisfactory treatment of hookworm infection is by tetrachloroethylene, alone or combined with chenopodium oil. This combination is frequently used also for removing tapeworms, especially if male fern has proved unsuccessful. It is given in a single dose of 1–3 ml. (15–45 min.) often in *Capsules*.

Many other substances have been used as anthelmintics. Of these, *Hexylresorcinol* (p. 307) deserves special mention. Though not the most powerful anthelmintic against any particular species of worm, it is one of the most valuable general anthelmintics as it is active against many different worms. It is especially valuable in mixed infections or when other more specific anthelmintics are contra-indicated. It is a local irritant and is therefore usually given as **Hexylresorcinol Pills**, U.S.P., 1 Gm., but the systemic toxicity of it is low.

SCHISTOSOMES (BILHARZIA)

The worms previously considered inhabit primarily the lumen of the intestine, and are readily accessible to drugs. Some worms, now to be dealt with, inhabit the tissues of the host and present a more difficult problem.

Diseases due to different species of flukes, e.g. *Schistosoma haematobium* and *Schistosoma mansoni* are widely distributed, especially in Egypt and South America and cause much disability. The adult flukes inhabit mainly pelvic veins and the female discharges large numbers of ova, each possessing a spike. These eggs pass through the mucous membrane of the bladder (*S. haematobium*) or of the rectum (*S. mansoni*) and, due to the trauma so caused, produce either haematuria or blood in the stools.

Of the remedies which are effective in stopping the passage of live ova, antimony compounds (p. 69) have already been mentioned. Lucanthone is a yellow synthetic compound readily absorbed when taken by mouth—a great advantage with some populations who resent injections, which are necessary with antimony compounds. This compound effectively stops reproduction of the parasite and may kill the parent flukes, so that, apart from reinfection, no relapses occur.

FILARIAE

There are several types of filariae, a nematode worm, which cause disease in tropical and subtropical countries. The adult worms inhabit the lymphatics of the abdomen, legs, external genitals, &c., causing a variety of obstructive symptoms depending on their distribution, e.g. lymphangitis or elephantiasis. The most important parasite is *Wuchereria* (*Filaria*) *bancrofti*, the female worm being 3–4 inches in length and the male about half as long. They shed embryos, microfilariae, in thousands into the blood stream but the presence of these causes little inconvenience. The disease is conveyed from one human being to another by biting insects. Antimony compounds, such as *Stibophen*, B.P., U.S.P., have been used with some success for killing the worms, but *Diethylcarbamazine Citrate*, B.P., U.S.P. (Hetrazan), a piperazine derivative introduced in 1947, has proved the most successful remedy. This compound has no effect on microfilariae *in vitro* but affects them in the blood so that they are taken up by the phagocytic reticulo-endothelial cells in the liver and rapidly vanish from the circulation. It is possible that the adult worms are killed also, or at least prevented from reproducing, because, after adequate treatment, microfilariae may not reappear in the blood even after 12 months. Hetrazan has a low toxicity but may produce nausea and, especially in heavy infections, allergic reactions due to liberation of products of destruction of the parasites, e.g. fever and itching. It is given orally, in doses of 0·15–0·5 G. daily B.P.; 2 mg. per kg. three times daily U.S.P.

INSECTICIDES AND INSECT REPELLENTS

Compared with their vast importance as vectors of diseases, insects are relatively unimportant as direct pathogenic agents, but two common ailments come under the latter category.

SCABIES

In this disease a minute insect (*Sarcoptes scabiei*) burrows into the skin and there deposits its eggs. This causes irritation and itch.

Ointment of Sulphur, B.P. (10 per cent.), rubbed into the skin kills the insect. This is usually done for three or four nights and then discontinued for, if applied longer, sulphur may cause irritation of the skin and dermatitis.

Benzyl Benzoate, B.P., U.S.P., a colourless oily liquid or crystals, insoluble in water, affords a more rapid and cleanly method of treating scabies than sulphur ointment. It is usually applied as a 10–30 per cent. emulsion. The B.P. has an official *Application* for this purpose.

PEDICULOSIS

Even in countries where they do not act as transmitters of diseases, pediculi (lice) can hardly be described as ideal fellow-travellers. Their unwelcome attentions produce ill health, owing to itch, discomfort, and sometimes associated dermatitis. The eggs attached for example to the hairs are more difficult to kill than the adult pediculi. Many remedies have been used, among the most successful being *Dicophane*, B.P., *Chloropheno-thane*, U.S.P., applied to the scalp as an emulsion. It kills the lice and its action lasts long enough to kill the young as they hatch.

Owing to the increasing recognition of the importance of insects as agents for the transmission and causation of disease both in animals and in plants, a vast amount of research has been devoted in recent years to the discovery of insecticides and new ones are constantly being produced. Here only those which are of established value for human disease can be mentioned.

INSECT REPELLENTS

Infections like malaria or typhus, which are conveyed to man and other animals by insect bites, cannot occur if the insects are prevented from biting. Substances which ward off insects are called insect repellents. Oil of citronella has a reputation for this but more efficient non-odorous synthetic compounds have been introduced in recent years. *Dimethyl Phthalate*, U.S.P., is used especially against mosquitoes. Applied to exposed parts, it is effective for a few hours, but its action may be prolonged for many hours by special devices, such as the use of veils impregnated with it. *Dibutyl Phthalate*, B.P., is used against mites and ticks and has a more prolonged action.

INSECTICIDES

Dicophane, B.P., *Chlorophenothane*, U.S.P., (DDT), is dichlorodiphenyl-trichloroethane, a colourless, insoluble synthetic insecticide. This substance, developed by Müller in

Switzerland in 1939, is soluble in organic solvents which, on evaporation, leave it as an adherent, weather-resistant crystal. It is a contact poison to insects, being absorbed by penetration of the exo-skeleton as well as in food. It is also toxic to mammals, fish, birds, but is seldom absorbed in quantity. Despite the appearance of many strains of flies resistant to DDT it has played an immense part in reducing the incidence of, or, in suitable districts, entirely eliminating the malarial vector *Anopheles*. It is effective in dusts or emulsions against other vectors—lice (typhus), fleas (plague), ticks (scrub typhus), tsetse (trypanosomiasis), &c., and has been broadcast over vast areas of the earth's surface.

Gamma Benzene Hexachloride, B.P., U.S.P., is practically insoluble in water. It is highly lethal to the same sorts of insects as is dicophane and like it is liable to give rise to resistant strains. It may be applied as a dust or spray to wide areas and inside buildings, and as a 1 per cent. emulsion to the body to eradicate lice, scabies, &c. It has been of great value in controlling *Anopheles*.

The development of strains of insects which have acquired resistance to modern insecticides is giving public-health authorities much concern. The number of important insect species which have given evidence of resistance to insecticides has risen to 37 in 1956 as compared with 13 in 1950, and only one in 1946 (W.H.O. report). Houseflies, cockroaches, lice, and anopheles, among other insects, have developed resistance in certain districts. It may reach a high degree, one species of larva in Trinidad being now 1,000 times as resistant to DDT as an untreated larval population. Resistance is acquired in different ways, the main cause of DDT resistance in the housefly being an increased rate of detoxification.

APPENDIX

AIDS TO DIAGNOSIS

THERE are a number of substances which are used for the information which they yield as to the functional or structural state of organs. Such substances are hardly to be classified as drugs since they are not used strictly as therapeutic agents but, as they are included in the pharmacopoeias, they are discussed here.

They may perhaps be classified best according to whether they measure function or aid direct observation of what would otherwise be difficult or impossible to see.

MEASUREMENT OF FUNCTION

(a) Renal function

Indigo Carmine, B.P., *Sodium Indigotindisulfonate*, U.S.P., is an odourless, blue, crystalline powder with a saline taste, which is readily soluble in water but is precipitated from solution by the addition of sodium chloride. It may be given slowly intravenously in a sterile 0·4 per cent. solution in a dose of 8–16 mg. or more. The urine appears discoloured at the ureteric orifices in 5–20 minutes' time, which is of value in helping to locate the openings in cases of difficulty when employing the cystoscope. The concentration in the urine after a given time interval gives a measure of renal clearance. *Phenolsulphonphthalein*, B.P., U.S.P., is a red crystalline powder which is soluble one part in 1,300 of water or one in 550 of alcohol. The dose by intramuscular or intravenous injection is 6 mg. It is given after some 400 ml. of water on an otherwise empty stomach. The urine is collected at stated intervals and the percentage of the dye which has been excreted in a given time estimated by comparison of the colour of the urine, when made alkaline, with standards. *Methylene Blue*, B.P., is a dark greenish crystalline powder which is soluble and may be sterilized. The dose is

60–300 mg. If 1 ml. or more of 5 per cent. solution is injected intramuscularly the urine becomes green in 30 minutes and the intensity of colour increases for 4 hours. It is generally considered to be inferior to indigo carmine.

Urea, B.P., U.S.P., forms colourless, soluble crystals with a saline taste. As mentioned (p. 26) it is a saline diuretic, for which purpose the U.S.P. recommends a dosage of 8 Gm. taken 1–5 times per day. When taken by mouth in solution it is excreted in the urine and the concentration, measured at hourly intervals should be not less than 2 per cent. A single dose B.P. is 5–15 G.

(b) Liver function

Sodium Benzoate, B.P., U.S.P., is a soluble white crystalline powder with a sweetish taste. It is mentioned in the U.S.P. as an antifungal agent and used in compounding certain syrups. It is included in the B.P. in a dose of 0·3–2 G. because of its use in Quick's Test of hepatic function. If 1·77 G. of sodium benzoate in 20 ml. sterile solution are injected intravenously the healthy liver will conjugate it as glucuronide and it will be excreted in the urine quantitatively in 1 hour, thus providing a ready measure of the detoxicating power of that organ. *Sulfobromophthalein Sodium Injection*, U.S.P., is a colourless sterile solution of 50 mg. per ml. of the compound. The dose is 5 mg./kg. weight injected intravenously. This substance is excreted rapidly in the bile and the rate of clearance from plasma may be measured quite readily and provides a measure of liver function.

(c) Gastric function

The use of histamine in determining the ability of the stomach to secrete acid has been mentioned (p. 182).

AIDS TO DIRECT OBSERVATION

(a) Blood volume

Evans Blue, U.S.P., is a hygroscopic green-blue powder which may be injected intravenously in a dose of 5 ml. of 0·5 per cent. solution (25 mg.). The dye is bound to plasma protein and thus diluted according to the volume of blood. Samples are withdrawn at a fixed time and the concentration measured, from which information the blood volume can be calculated.

(b) The visualization of corneal defects

Fluorescein Sodium, B.P., U.S.P., is an orange-red hygroscopic powder. Instilled into the conjunctival sac in a sterile 2 per cent. solution it stains any defect of the surface of the cornea and thus renders it visible.

(c) Visualization of the alimentary canal

The use of **Barium Sulphate**, B.P., U.S.P., which is insoluble and unabsorbed, in conjunction with X-ray photography or screening, to render visible the anatomical state of the alimentary canal has been mentioned (p. 176). This radio-opaque contrast medium may be given as a thick suspension by mouth (barium swallow) or as an enema.

(d) Visualization of the renal or biliary tracts and of body cavities

Iodine, being an element of high atomic weight and great density is relatively opaque to X-rays. Various preparations are used in conjunction with X-ray photography either by direct injection or instillation into body cavities to enable them to be seen (e.g. bronchography) or to show up an organ during the process of excretion and concentration, e.g. in the bile or urine (cholecystography, urography).

The compounds used are of two types: (1) water-soluble organic iodine compounds such as **Iodoxyl**, B.P., which is given intravenously in the form of the official **Injection**; **Iodophthalein**, B.P., U.S.P., which may be given by mouth or by injection and **Iodopyracet Injection**, U.S.P. These are used to delineate the gall bladder or the renal system after excretion, or the vascular bed, &c., for angiography. (2) water-insoluble organic iodine compounds or iodinated vegetable oils such as **Injection of Iodised Oil**, B.P. U.S.P., **Iodoalphionic Acid**, U.S.P., and **Iopanoic Acid**, U.S.P., are mainly used for cholecystography after oral administration, but the oil may be injected into cavities such as fistulae, the bronchi, uterus, &c.

Two types of toxic reaction, both in the nature of an anaphylactic response, may be unexpectedly encountered. The first is a collapse of the patient associated with asthma and urticaria, the second is equally alarming and is a 'nitritoid crisis'—acute circulatory failure.

INDEX

PRINTED IN
GREAT BRITAIN
AT THE
UNIVERSITY PRESS
OXFORD
BY
CHARLES BATEY
PRINTER
TO THE
UNIVERSITY